'At last we have Ernst's book available to us. This book is a gift! A beautiful accompaniment to enrich the gentle healing energetic teachings of Marma Therapy. A life-changing treatment with its roots in ancient Ayurveda and its future in modern therapy. Marma Therapy has remarkable healing ability. This book is beautifully illustrated and gives a clear and highly informative description of the treatment philosophy, procedure and the benefits that can be achieved. Thank you for sharing this gift – it will enrich the healing capacity of many therapists. I highly recommend this book and the teachings of Ernst Schrott.'

*– Beverley Higham, aromatherapist and author*

'What impresses me most whenever I have Sukshma Marma Therapy is that something so gentle and so precise can have such a profound healing effect. Amazing how profoundly effective this gentleness is. Just fantastic.'

*– Princess Ursula Blücher von Wahlstatt*

'Sukshma Marma Therapy® is a simple, powerful, safe procedure that anyone can learn and benefit from. It brings together the ancient wisdom of Ayurveda with essential oils, gentle touch and pure intention. In this book, Dr. Schrott presents a simple and practical guide so that anyone can take the first steps to learning this profound practice for use on themselves and on others.'

*– Jonathan Hinde MA (Oxon), aromatherapy writer, Director of Oshadhi Ltd, and teacher of Transcendental Meditation*

'This wonderful book represents the product of 30 years' work by some of the greatest minds in the field of mind-body and consciousness. They have revived the almost-lost Ayurvedic knowledge of the therapeutic treatment of Marma points and made it accessible to anyone anywhere in the world. Marmas are the delicate, subtle points in the physiology where consciousness and matter are most intimately connected. By gentle touch the mind and body can be treated. I highly recommend this unique book to anyone who is interested in promoting life in the direction of perfect health.'

*– Dr. Elizabeth L. Young, General Practitioner, London*

'I had a neural lesion on my face with no sensation in the right side for about 30 years. I was invited to participate in a workshop session and the result was the restoration of sensation in my face. I knew then that this is one of the most powerful tools that we in the health sector can give to ourselves and our patients - an efficient, clean and gentle treatment method. In 30 years as a medical doctor, I never saw anything like this. Thanks Ernst.'

*– Guilherme Oberlaender MD, Brazil*

'Training with Ernst has given me a new Angel touch method to bring the body back to balance. Who wants to run their life by fear and old traumas? This is a book to gain your freedom and happiness.'

*– Gudrun Jonsson, Biopath, Reflexologist and author of* Gut Reaction

First published by Mosaik Verlag, Munich, Germany in 2009

English language edition first published in 2016
by Singing Dragon
an imprint of Jessica Kingsley Publishers
73 Collier Street
London N1 9BE, UK
and
400 Market Street, Suite 400
Philadelphia, PA 19106, USA

www.singingdragon.com



**Library of Congress Cataloging in Publication Data**

Schrott, Ernst G., 1951-
[Marmatherapie. English]
Marma therapy / Dr. Ernst Schrott, Dr. J. Ramanuja Raju, and Stefan Schrott.
pages cm
Includes index.
ISBN 978-1-84819-296-6 (alk. paper)
1. Medicine, Ayurvedic. 2. Acupuncture points. I. Raju, J. Ramanuja. II. Schrott, Stefan. III. Title.
R127.2.S3713 2016
610--dc23

2015031152

**British Library Cataloguing in Publication Data**

A CIP catalogue record for this book is available from the British Library

ISBN 978 1 84819 296 6
eISBN 978 0 85701 246 3

Printed and bound in China

# Marma Therapy

DR. ERNST SCHROTT, DR. J. RAMANUJA RAJU
AND STEFAN SCHROTT

Translated by Marek Lorys

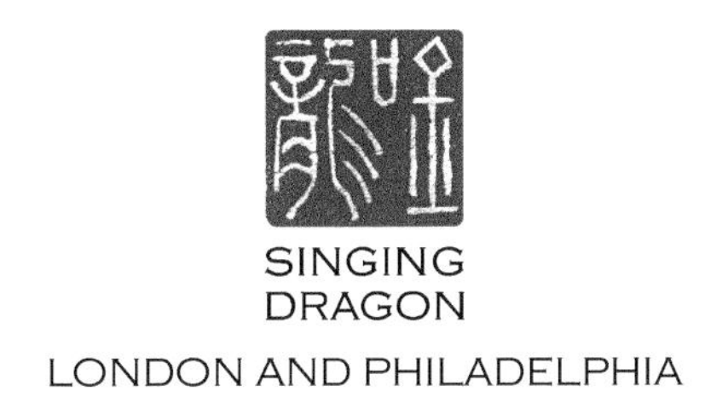

SINGING
DRAGON
LONDON AND PHILADELPHIA

# Contents

Preface . . . . . 6

## Gentle Therapy for the Energy Points

### Marmas and the Healing Power of Your Hands. . . . . 8

Prana, the healing energy . . . . . 9
Sensors for finer perception and power centres . . . 9
The primordial sound of creation vibrates in the Marmas . . . . . 9
Cosmic switchboards . . . . . 10
How many Marmas are there? . . . . . 10

### The Order and Structure of the Marmas. . . . . 11

The five administrative districts of the seven main energy centres . . . . . 12
The entire body is reflected in your hands and feet . . . . . 13
The number 108 is significant. . . . . 13
The Marmas and the moon. . . . . 14
The three super-ministries . . . . . 15

### Ayurvedic Principles and Marmas . . . . . 16

Marmas and the three Doshas . . . . . 16
The three Doshas briefly characterized . . . . . 17
Subdoshas – five subtypes of the bioregulators. . . . 17

### The Marma Point – Principal Control Centre . . . . 18

The Marma House. . . . . 19
Classification of Marmas by the consequences of injury. . . . . 21
Differences between Marmas according to the predominant tissue type . . . . . 21

## Types of Marma Therapy

### Different Treatment Methods. . 24

Proper touch heals . . . . . 25
Applying ointments, herbs and oils to a Marma point. . . . . 25
Rasayanas – rejuvenation remedies of Ayurveda . . . 26
Oil bath on a Marma . . . . . 27
Treatment through the five senses . . . . . 28
Marmas respond to sound and music . . . . . 29
Marmas and meditation . . . . . 30
Yoga, Mudras and breathing exercises . . . . . 30
The Yagya ceremony . . . . . 30

## Treatment Techniques

### General Rules for Marma Treatment . . . . . 32

Preparing for a treatment. . . . . 32
The importance of pressure in massage . . . . . 32
The strokes . . . . . 33
The number of massage strokes – the 1–3–5–7 format . . . . . 34
The significance and effects of fingers and the palm of the hand. . . . . 35
Marmas inside and out – a harmonious partnership. . . . . 36
Choosing the right oil . . . . . 36
The order of treatment of individual Marmas . . . . 38
Tips for self-treatment . . . . . 39
Tips for partner treatment . . . . . 40

## Marmas: Meaning and Treatment


### Marmas on the Arms and Legs . 42

The Marmas between the fingers – Kshipra . . . . .44
The heart of the hand – Talahridaya . . . . . . . . . .46
The wrist Marma – Manibandha . . . . . . . . . . . .48
The forearm Marma – Indrabasti . . . . . . . . . . .50
The elbow Marma – Kurpara . . . . . . . . . . . . . .52
Further Marmas on the arm . . . . . . . . . . . . . .54
The Marma between the toes – Kshipra . . . . . . .56
The heart of the foot – Talahridaya . . . . . . . . . .58
The ankle Marma – Gulpha . . . . . . . . . . . . . .60
The calf Marma – Indrabasti . . . . . . . . . . . . . .62
The knee Marma – Janu . . . . . . . . . . . . . . . . .64
Further Marmas on the leg . . . . . . . . . . . . . . .66

### The Seven Mahamarmas and Marmas of the Chest. . . . . . . . 68

The pelvic floor Marma – Guda . . . . . . . . . . . .70
The bladder Marma – Basti . . . . . . . . . . . . . . .72
The navel Marma – Nabhi . . . . . . . . . . . . . . .74
The great heart Marma – Hridaya . . . . . . . . . . .76
Additional Marmas in the chest area . . . . . . . . . .78

### Marmas of the Pelvis and Back . 80

The Marmas of the pelvis along the lumbar spine . .82
The large Marma of the back – Brihati . . . . . . . . .84
The Marma of the shoulder blade – Amsaphalaka . .86
The shoulder–neck Marma – Amsa . . . . . . . . . .88

### Marmas of the Head and Neck . 90

The neck Marmas – Nila, Manya and Sira Matrika . .92
The eye Marmas – Avarta and Apanga . . . . . . . .94
The ear Marma – Vidhura . . . . . . . . . . . . . . .96
The neck Marma – Krikatika . . . . . . . . . . . . . .98
The temple Marmas – Shankha and Utkshepa . . . 100
The palate Marma – Shringataka . . . . . . . . . . . 102
The third eye – Sthapani . . . . . . . . . . . . . . . 104
The crown Marma – Simanta . . . . . . . . . . . . . 106
The crown Marma – Adhipati . . . . . . . . . . . . . 108


## Mudras and Marmas


### Conscious Gestures Lead Inwards . . . . . . . . . . . . . . . .111

Attention improves the effect . . . . . . . . . . . . . 111
Each Mudra has its grace . . . . . . . . . . . . . . . 111
Understanding the effects of the Mudras . . . . . . 112
Mudras and Doshas . . . . . . . . . . . . . . . . . . 113
Mudras manifest Marmas . . . . . . . . . . . . . . . 113
Finger Mudras . . . . . . . . . . . . . . . . . . . . . 114


## Yoga and Marmas


### Strengthening the Marmas with Properly Executed Yoga Asanas . 120

Yoga is not gymnastics . . . . . . . . . . . . . . . . 121
Your well-being is the measure of success . . . . . . 121
Remain relaxed throughout . . . . . . . . . . . . . . 121

### The Effect of Yoga Postures on the Marmas . . . . . . . . . . . .122

Diamond posture – Vajrasana . . . . . . . . . . . . . 122
Sitting forward bend – Janu Sirasana . . . . . . . . . 122
Half spinal twist – Matsyendrasana . . . . . . . . . . 122
A simple practice set for all Marmas . . . . . . . . . 123
Pranayama – gentle alternate nostril breathing . . . 126


## Marma Therapy for Everyday Complaints


### Supporting Self-healing with Marmas and Ayurveda . . . . . .128

Nervous disorders of the heart . . . . . . . . . . . . 130
Sleep disorders . . . . . . . . . . . . . . . . . . . . . 131
Headache and migraine . . . . . . . . . . . . . . . . 132
Complete back treatment . . . . . . . . . . . . . . . 134
Treatment of the upper back . . . . . . . . . . . . . 136
Treatment of the chest Marmas . . . . . . . . . . . . 136
Treatment of the 15 Marmas of the moon . . . . . 138

Further Reading and Useful Addresses . . . . . . . 140
Index . . . . . . . . . . . . . . . . . . . . . . . . . . 142
Acknowledgements . . . . . . . . . . . . . . . . . . 146
About the Authors . . . . . . . . . . . . . . . . . . . 147

# Preface

It must have been a fortunate coincidence that the chambermaid in the South Indian hotel where I was staying happened to be singing one of her soulful songs as she worked. She was one of those innocent souls you probably find only in this country, which is steeped in tradition and respect for God's creation. Alongside her job she was studying traditional Indian voice, which she now intoned with deep devotion for the Divine and its manifold expressions. The melodies she sang immediately touched the heart, uplifting one's very Being to a finer, divine realm.

Sound and melody – the eternal music of nature – are, according to Ayurveda, the subtle basis of the human physiology. The melodies of the heart vibrate in the Marmas and fill them with happiness and peace. It was this experience, later followed by the practical application of Marma Therapy on our patients, which confirmed in my mind the great value and undiscovered potential of the Marmas. Marmas are vital points and energy fields which are essential for health, happiness and a long life in spiritual fulfilment.

Currently, Marma Therapy is used in just a very limited manner in traditional Indian natural medicine. Furthermore the therapy as currently practised generally concentrates less on the energy field and consciousness of the Marma point and more on the physical structures which are included in massages. This kind of treatment has many similarities with muscle, tendon and trigger point massage in Western physiotherapy.

In this book we introduce a very gentle technique that we have developed for treating Marmas. It brings inner tranquillity, and therefore has its primary effect on the level of consciousness and then on the body and its organs. For this reason we call it sukshma, or gentle, Marma treatment. In Sukshma Marma Therapy, the main attention is on the energetic aspects of the Marma points: the field of consciousness of the Marmas.

Dr. Ernst Schrott

# Gentle Therapy for the Energy Points

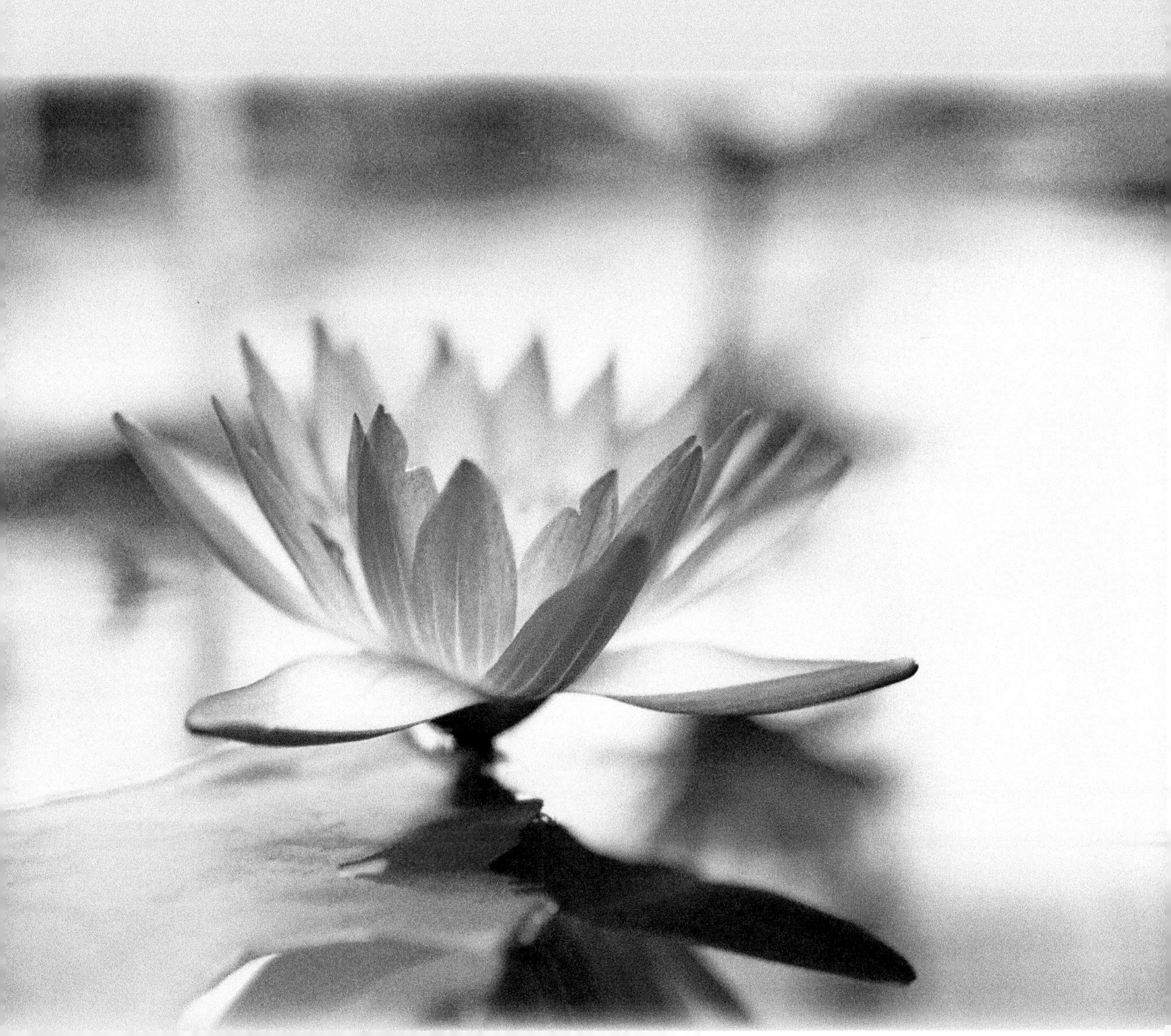

# Marmas and the Healing Power of Your Hands

## 'Marma is the Seat of Life.'

*SUSHRUTA SAMHITA*, CLASSIC TEXTBOOK OF AYURVEDIC MEDICINE

Marma Therapy – the art of treating specific vital points on the human body – is one of the greatest healing secrets of Ayurveda. It can be used to detoxify, strengthen and revitalize the body, for rejuvenation and relaxation or to release blocked energy. Using these subtle energy points we can stimulate the function of the internal organs, promote self-healing and harmonize mind and body. We can improve eyesight, balance the digestive system, alleviate headaches, reduce tension and alleviate or cure many other everyday complaints.

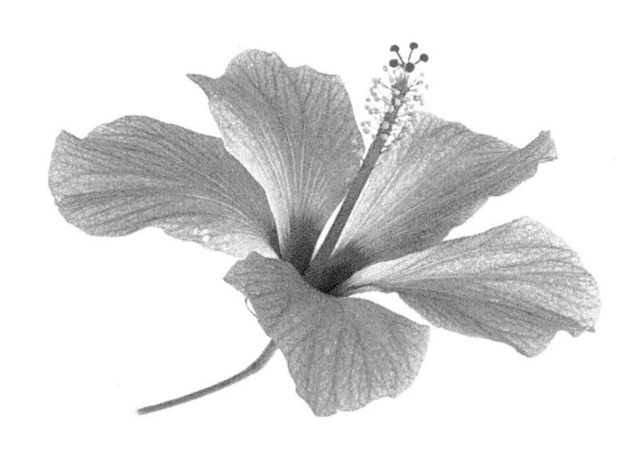

Marma Therapy covers a wide spectrum of applications, from simple self-treatment to elaborate clinical therapy which requires extensive medical experience and specially trained therapists. As an independent form of therapy it is practised almost exclusively in South India. But, in general, almost all Ayurvedic treatment includes Marmas as the key points of the body and mind: in massage and oil application, herbal and heat packs and cleansing treatments. Even meditation with mantras, the wearing of gemstones, treatment with light and colour or healing scents aim to use the healing potential of specific Marmas. The gentle method of the Marma treatment that we present in this book is especially applicable for self or partner treatment. It requires only a few basic skills, a degree of physical sensitivity and, above all, delight in touch, massage and well-being.

Sukshma Marma Therapy® (SMT, Sukha Marma Therapy® or Marma Protection Therapy) was developed on the basis of traditional Vedic knowledge and classical Ayurvedic texts, as well as many years of study and research, supplemented by practical and clinical experience and oral Marma traditions. Thus, not all concepts discussed in this book will be found in classical Marma literature.

## Prana, the healing energy

Marma Therapy, in its essence, is treatment that involves healing with our hands (in German: Be*hand*lung). However, we should not consider ourselves miracle healers because the healing power of hands is dormant in all of us. This subtle energy flowing out of the palm and the fingers is physiological, natural and essential for life. Without it, life would not exist. In Ayurveda, we call this special healing energy *Prana*. Prana is the first vibration, the first mover that transforms the silence of the universe into manifest life and it is that which exists as vital breath, an expression of the consciousness of all living beings. This Prana flows through all *Nadis*, the finest energy channels in the body, and resides in a concentrated form in its energy points, the Marmas.

Our hands are full of such Marmas, large and small, and these give us the sensitivity to feel mentally and physically, informing the way we move our hands and the way we touch. Prana in the hands allows us to give love. It is the power by which we naturally treat and also heal ourselves and others in everyday life.

## Sensors for finer perception and power centres

Marmas are subtle, intelligent and very powerful control points in the mind and body. In these vital points on the surface of the body we find not only condensed information about physiology, physical organs and systems, but also the content of consciousness and emotions. However, Marmas do not only operate within, they are also our antennae to the outside world, sensors for more subtle perception. They let us sense or see the aura of a person. They sense the future and share it with us, maybe only as a vague, queasy feeling in the stomach, in *Nabhi*, the navel Marma, if something bad threatens, something that we cannot put into words, simply a subtle notion. Or they give us insight and foresight, a clear vision of the future. The master Marma for this when it is fully developed is the 'third eye', *Sthapani*. Marmas are the power centres of the body, comparable to power places on earth at certain energetic interfaces on our planet.

## The primordial sound of creation vibrates in the Marmas

Man, nature and cosmos are considered as one in Vedic medicine: it recognizes the myriad interactions between the individual and the environment. Diagnosis and therapy therefore include the living environment, social life, the external forces of nature, the influence of the time of day and seasons, and even the cosmic influence of planets and galaxies. The Marmas are central to these interactions. The phases of the moon alter the energy level of the Marmas in the same way that they affect the tides. The planets in the solar system affect the main Marmas at the centre of the body with their cosmic qualities, and their qualities strengthen and weaken in a cyclical way. Marma Therapy is therefore one of the most intelligent healing approaches of Vedic medicine and also the most delicate because in the Marmas we touch consciousness, Veda and the cosmos.

## Cosmic switchboards

Marmas are the junction points between mind, body and consciousness. More than that, they are the seams between the cosmos and the individual. The great Vedic scholar of our time, Maharishi Mahesh Yogi (d. 2008), described them as cosmic switchboards, the human organism's cosmic control panels. In the Marmas, the primordial sounds of the Vedas are alive. Each Marma is like a special instrument with its own individual sound in an orchestra that plays the symphony of life. The Marmas communicate through a complex system of innumerable Nadis, literally 'sound channels'. The ancient Vedic texts, the earliest *Upanishads*, speak of 72,000 such energy channels that emanate from the heart and contain the flow of Prana, the vital breath.

## How many Marmas are there?

In the *Sushruta Samhita*, Ayurvedic medicine's textbook of surgery, 107 key energy points are listed. These form the basic framework for a regulating and balancing treatment with oils, ointments, essential oils, specific massage techniques and a number of other applications. Beyond that, there are thousands of additional, smaller control points distributed over the body. The ancient Vedic martial art which is still practised in South India in the Kalari tradition (page 21) recognizes 365 points. Traditional Chinese Medicine (TCM) records a similar number. This knowledge has developed from acupuncture, a form of treatment which has successfully treated and cured diseases for thousands of years. The ancient Chinese doctors called these points, literally, 'forwarding gate'. Marma, a Sanskrit word, means 'sensitive', 'hidden' and also 'vital point'.

### THE VEDA

Veda is the primordial sound of creation, pure knowledge, the organizing intelligence on which all life is based. Veda is the genuine perception of the great seers and sages, the 'Maharishis' of the Vedic era. Thousands of years ago, deep within themselves, they perceived the laws of nature within their own consciousness in the silence of meditation. They experienced themselves as one with the universe, connected to everything in the eternal existence of pure Being. This Being, the silent intelligence of nature, the Veda, they described as the common and universal source of all order of nature and of life itself.

# The Order and Structure of the Marmas

HIERARCHICAL UNFOLDMENT OF THE MARMAS

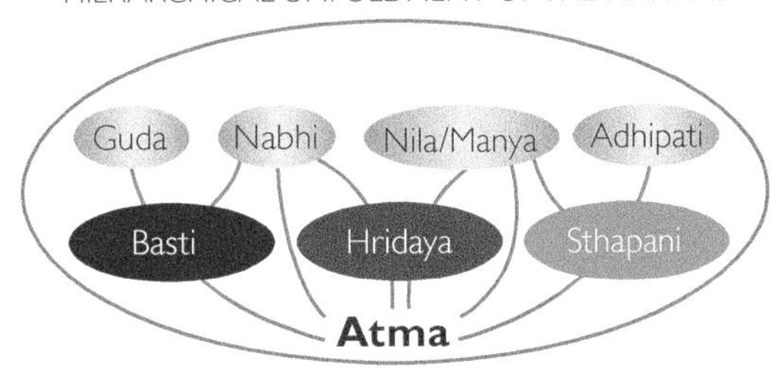


*The Self or Atma, made of pure, undivided consciousness, expresses itself as first three and then four more central Marmas. These are the control centres for all other Marmas in the body.*

If we look more closely at the Marmas, we see a logical system, a distinct hierarchical structure (see above). This can be compared to a government-like system with various ministries, divisions with specialists, local representatives, local government offices, and an absolute ruler at the top. This ruler is our Self – in Ayurveda called Atma. It is the primary Marma, underlying all the others. All the other Marmas spring forth from Atma and are all connected to it.

In the first stage of manifestation, **three** great Mahamarmas can be located in the middle of the body: Sthapani, Hridaya and Basti, which have their seats of power at the head, heart and abdomen (see opposite). These three are supported by four other principal Marmas, which are also centrally located on the body and are arranged alongside the first three Marmas. These are the root Marma, Guda, at the anus; the navel Marma, Nabhi; the neck Marmas Nila and Manya; and finally, 'the supreme ruler', Adhipati, sitting on the top of the head.

All the other Marmas are grouped around these **seven** major centres and are subject to their dominion. As we will see later, these centrally located Marmas are connected to the seven Chakras of Yoga teaching (see page 81). They are related to the seven body tissue types or *Dhatus*, as described in Ayurveda, to the different subdivisions of the Ayurvedic bioregulators, or *Doshas* (see below), to the seven layers of the aura and to the seven main planets in Vedic astrology.

THE PRINCIPAL SEAT OF THE THREE DOSHAS AND THE THREE MAHAMARMAS

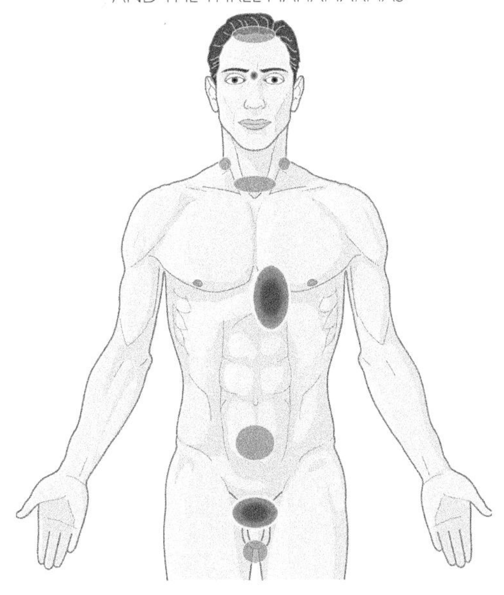

Kapha: *Head*
Sthapani: *the forehead Marma, the head centre, the 'third eye', Rishi*
Pitta: *Solar plexus and chest*
Hridaya: *the heart Marma, Devata*
Vata: *Lower abdomen*
Basti: *the bladder Marma, Chhandas*

## The five administrative districts of the seven main energy centres

The figures below show schematically the administrative districts of the principal energy centres in the body. Each of them governs directly through a group of other Marmas in its locality and is also connected with all the central and peripheral power centres on the arms and legs. The five physiological regions, or main administrative areas, are anatomically divided into: pelvis, abdomen, chest, neck and head. These are the locations and main centres of the five expressions of Pranic energy: *Apana Vata* (Pelvis, Guda and Basti), *Samana Vata* (Nabhi), *Vyana Vata* (Hridaya), *Udana Vata* (Nila/Manya) and *Prana Vata* (Sthapani, Adhipati).

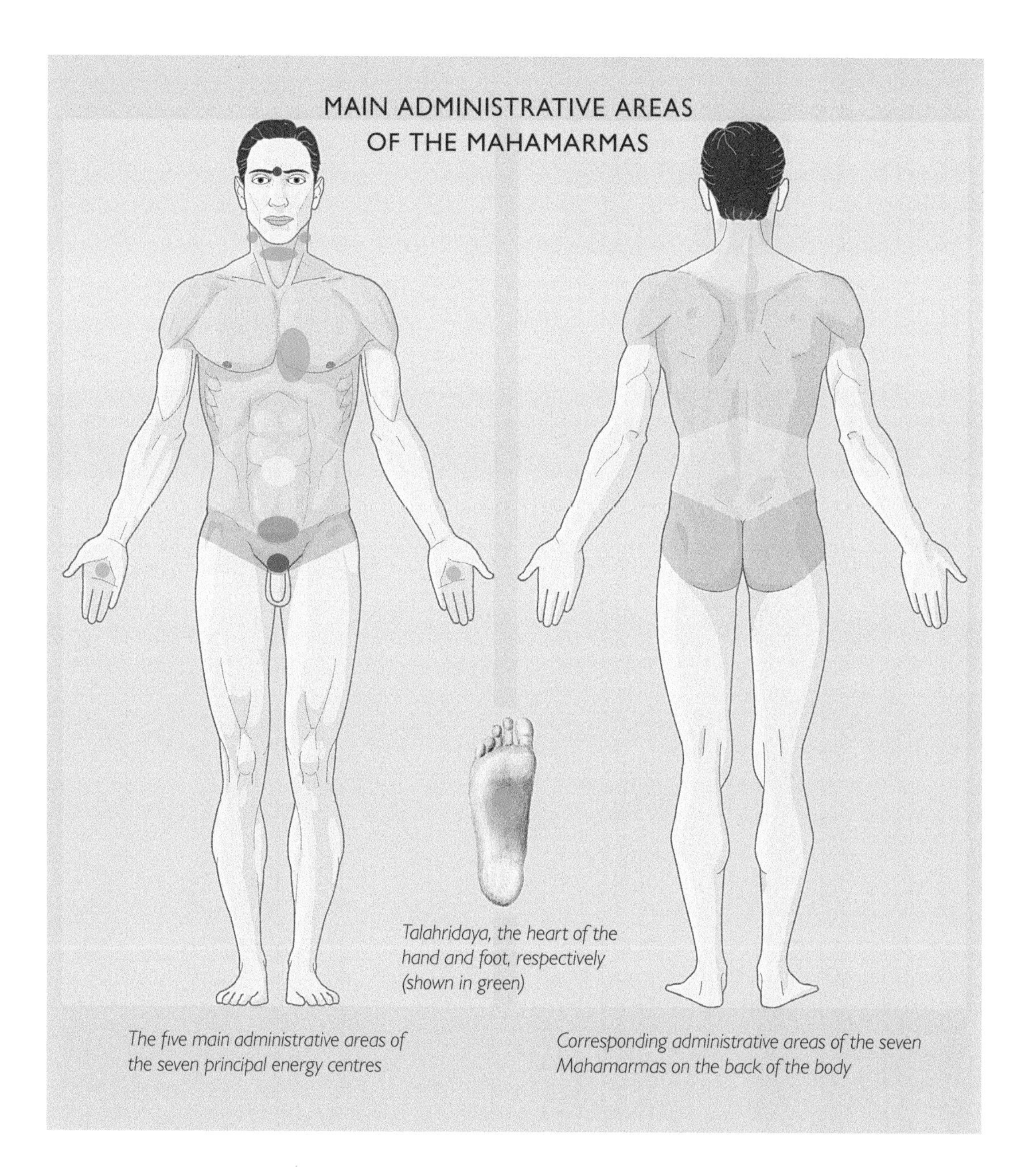


*Talahridaya, the heart of the hand and foot, respectively (shown in green)*

*The five main administrative areas of the seven principal energy centres*

*Corresponding administrative areas of the seven Mahamarmas on the back of the body*

## The entire body is reflected in your hands and feet

The Marmas in the hands and feet are representatives of the great Marmas in the centre of the body. The hand is like an outpost of the government, whose ministries are also represented here. The centre of the palm of the hand and the sole of the foot are the outposts of the heart Marma and the solar plexus. This Marma is tellingly named 'heart of the hand', Talahridaya (tala = hand, hridaya = heart). We will refer to it many times in the therapy part of the book because of its central role, just as the heart Marma itself is of great significance.

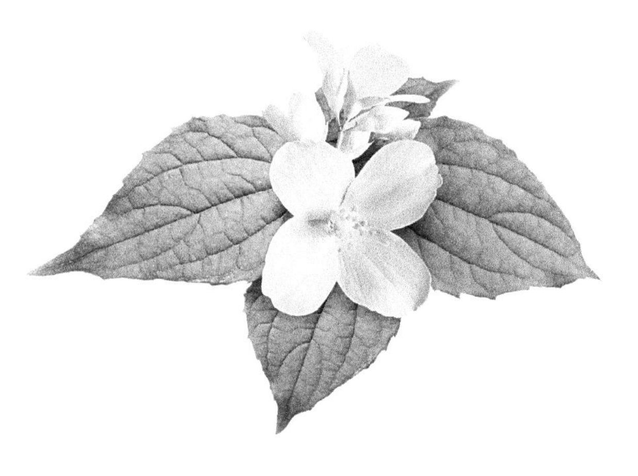

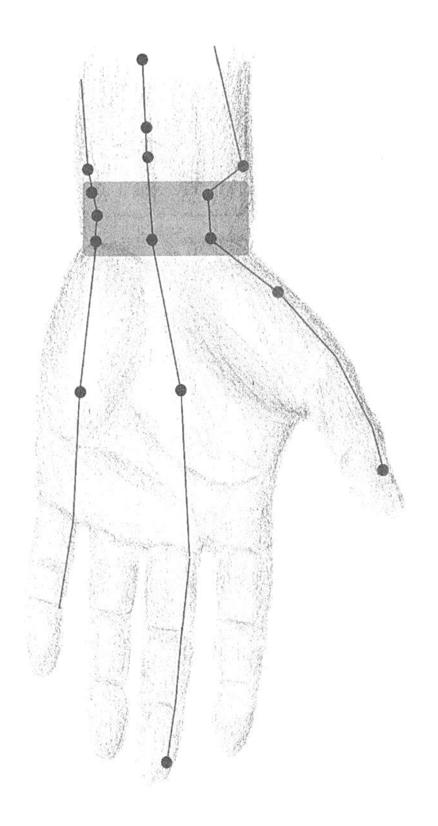

*There are small vital points along the energy lines described by TCM: the lung (thumb), pericardium (middle finger) and heart (little finger) meridians. These are controlled by the superordinate wrist Marma.*

## The number 108 is significant

If we include Atma, the Self, as the primordial Marma, we can count a total of 108 energy points. These are the main energy points out of a huge number of different energy points spread over the entire body. They coordinate countless other smaller vital points. The figure opposite shows an example of the wrist Marma *Manibandha*. Note that there are a number of small vital points along the meridians (some of which are described in South Indian Siddha medicine). Traditional Chinese Medicine (TCM) shows their precise location and connections and uses these as the basis for acupuncture. The wrist Marma is primary and coordinates their activity.

Since these main Marmas often cover relatively large areas (see page 11), it is easy to locate them – unlike the small vital points – and in treating them we simultaneously affect the smaller sub-Marmas and acupuncture points. This greatly simplifies our approach.

## The Marmas and the moon

There is a further remarkable correlation between the number of Marmas – 108 – and the moon! Our earth's satellite has a powerful influence on Prana, which is the essential energy of the Marmas and meridians. To understand this, we can think of a Marma as a lake of energy with tides that are affected by the moon. The deepest point is in its centre, *Bindu*, which is the central and most effective point of a Marma. Towards the shore, the Marma lake is shallower. As the moon waxes and increases in energy, this energy lake expands, and as it wanes the Marmas shrink again. During the 28-day cycle of a lunar month (astrologically; known as *Tithtis*), each Marma is sequentially charged with Pranic energy, starting with the Marmas on the feet (the right foot for men and the left foot for women – see also pages 138–139), rising above the waist to the head at the full moon. With the waning moon, Prana is reduced in the Marmas until the next new moon, when everything starts again.

During its journey through the starlit sky the moon passes through the constellations in 27 days. Western and Vedic astrology divide the ecliptic into 27 segments, known as lunar mansions or *Nakshatras*. (Incidentally, the 27 Nakshatras correspond to cell groups in the brain stem, clusters of neurons that have a wide range of functions and which are linked to the entire nervous system. These are also exactly 27 in number; see Nader 2001 in Further Reading and Useful Addresses.)

Each lunar mansion is also divided into four time periods, known as *Padas*, which have defined astrological characteristics, and we can assign one Marma to each Pada. The total number is thus four times 27, or 108 overall. If we include Atma, the Self, pure, undivided consciousness, as the primordial Marma, we get to the exact number of Marmas that Sushruta and other classical authors have described as being particularly significant.

### INFLUENCE OF THE MOON ON THE TIDES OF THE MARMAS

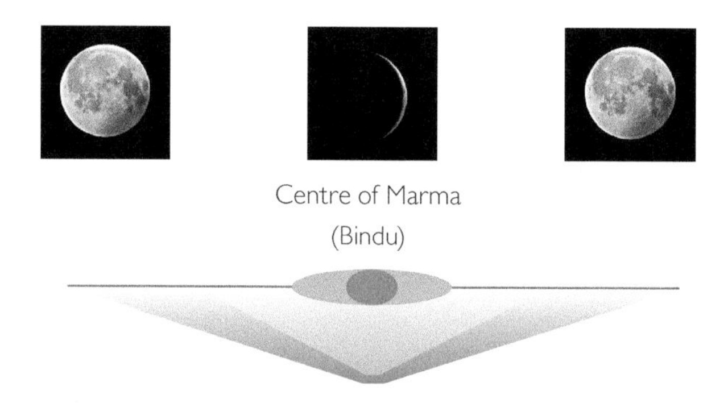


*The influence of the phases of the moon on the Marmas resembles the effect on tides: as the moon waxes, Prana increases in the Marmas and then, during the waning moon, pranic energy ebbs.*

## The three super-ministries

Let us look again at the first three major Marmas: these form the three main resonance or energy centres from which all the Nadis – the energy channels – emerge and connect to all the other Marmas. All meridians, or energy channels, run into and originate from them. They are like three super-ministries in one organized governmental system and are the primary residences of the most fundamental qualities of emotion and intelligence (see illustration on page 11). This is because Marmas constitute different expressions of consciousness in the body.

### 1. The Head Marma – Shiromarma

The whole head is a Marma. It has its own system of perception and carries a form of 'I' or individual consciousness. Its centre is the Marma of the 'third eye' – *Sthapani*. If we close our eyes, we find ourselves behind the eyes. Here we live as a kind of seeing awareness or, in the language of Ayurveda, as a *Rishi*. The head is the capital of the senses and mind. It is the seat of *analytical intelligence*.

### 2. The Heart Marma – Hridaya

The heart is regarded as the main residence of our soul. We point to it directly with our hand when we say 'me'. It is here that our *sentient* awareness resides. This Marma is a place of *emotional intelligence*, and it corresponds to *Devata*.

### 3. The Abdominal or Bladder Marma – Basti

In the abdominal Marma, *Basti*, we find a form of instinctive consciousness (*Chhandas*). Through this we connect with the earthly things in life, the premonitions and instincts, and also with the field of desire. The lower abdomen, with *Basti* as its energetic centre, is the seat of *archaic intelligence*, where the sense of basic trust, genetically predetermined automatic functions and primordial behaviour patterns all manifest.

These three major Marmas are closely connected with the three bioenergies of Ayurveda, the Doshas: *Vata*, *Pitta* and *Kapha* (see illustration on page 11).

### Everything is connected to everything

What can we conclude from this hierarchical arrangement of the Marmas? In terms of treatment there are several important considerations:

- if we treat one of those central and superior Marmas, then we also affect all the other Marmas around these big energy centres and in their area of influence
- if we treat a peripheral Marma, then we simultaneously treat the central Marma which is directly connected to it
- if we treat one Marma then we simultaneously treat all other Marmas. Nothing exists in isolation; everything is continuously interacting with everything else.

# Ayurvedic Principles and Marmas

There is a close relationship between Marmas and other Ayurvedic concepts and we will briefly mention them here, both because it helps to understand the function of the Marmas and because we will be referring to them when we come to the section on practice (page 41). If you would like to find out more about the terminology and concepts of Ayurvedic medicine, please see the Further Reading on pages 140–141.

## Marmas and the three Doshas

The three main Marmas are closely related to the three Doshas (bioregulators), which also have their principal seat in the same regions: Vata in the lower abdomen, Pitta in the solar plexus and heart area, and Kapha in the head (see page 11).

Doshas are like a triad (in the sense of three notes of a musical chord) for our personality. If they are well tuned and in harmony, then we feel healthy, happy, powerful and full of positive energy and enthusiasm. If, however, one Dosha is out of tune, like one string of an instrument, then disharmony is created and we feel discordant. With continued imbalance of the Doshas, physical and mental symptoms arise, resulting in what we finally call disease. The goal of all Ayurvedic therapies is therefore to maintain or restore balance in the Doshas. In this regard Marma Therapy is of particular significance and effectiveness, for the Doshas reside in the Marmas themselves and determine whether on the one hand they function perfectly or are blocked, or have defects or energetic weakness. The Doshas directly determine the nature and function of a Marma.

DYNAMIC BALANCE AND INTERDEPENDENCE OF THE DOSHAS

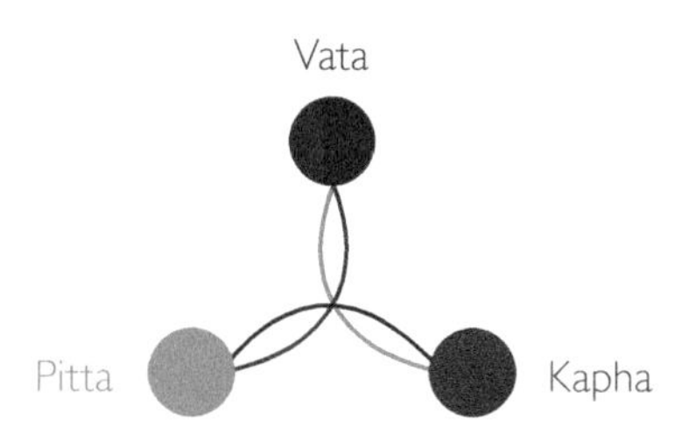


*The three Doshas are like a (musical) triad in the personality. When they are in balance, they create a unified togetherness, a mental and physical harmony. Health is an expression of the harmony of these psychophysical control principles.*

## The three Doshas briefly characterized

THE THREE DOSHAS AND THE FIVE ELEMENTS

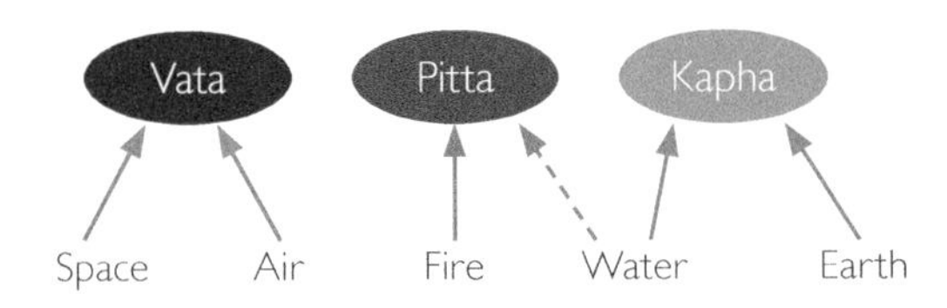


*The three Doshas and their properties are created and shaped by the five virtual life elements.*

**Vata** is the force that moves, changes and communicates. Any kind of animation is an expression of the activity of Vata: speaking, thinking, moving the fingers, the flow of breath, the rhythm of the heart, transportation of substances between the cells, communication with the environment and communication of the Marmas with each other. Marmas dominated by Vata will control all these functions. Vata is primarily associated with the nervous system. Its nature is lightness, like the air and space from which it is created.

**Pitta** produces energy, heat, transformation and metabolism. A person with a lot of Pitta has fire, energy and dynamism, and is purposeful, passionate and emotional. Pitta's element is fire, with also a little water. Marmas with dominant Pitta are responsible for metabolism, energy and heat production and they are the seat of emotions – for example, the heart Marma and also the heart of the hand, Talahridaya.

**Kapha** structures the body and is the basis of fluids and the solid parts of the body. People who by nature have more Kapha act in a calm, persistent, uniform and steady manner. They are mentally stable and physically heavy and strong. Earth and water form Kapha Dosha. Marmas with dominant Kapha mainly control Kapha functions.

## Subdoshas – five subtypes of the bioregulators

The three Doshas each contain five subfunctions, the Subdoshas. These will be explained as required as we discuss the different Marmas. The following are three brief examples:

- An important aspect of Vata is the function of excretion. One Subdosha of Vata is called *Apana* (*Apa-an* = 'downward movement'), and its main seat is in the Marmas located in the lower abdomen. *Apana* in *Guda*, the root Marma, regulates the elimination of faeces and wind. *Apana* in the bladder Marma – *Basti* – controls urination, menstruation and also the process of giving birth. *Apana* also controls letting go mentally, which is realized in these lowest energy centres.

- A Subdosha of Pitta, *Sadhaka*, has its seat in the heart, but also in the heart of the hand, *Talahridaya*, and in *Sthapani*, the 'heart of the head'. *Sthapani* is where we speculate and worry, and is therefore also an area where we experience the feelings of the heart. In principle, however, *Sadhaka* is present in all Marmas, because of the central role that the heart plays for all Marmas.

- *Prana Vata* is not only the energy and intelligence of the Marmas and Nadis, but also mental activity itself; that is, the process of thinking.

# The Marma Point – Principal Control Centre

What does a Marma point actually look like? Marmas are not anatomical structures – they are areas in the anatomy where consciousness connects with the body and coordinates its functions. Or to put it another way: Marmas are the places where intelligence transforms into matter, into the body. Each point is also a holographic image of all the Marmas – this means that all the information of one Marma is also present in all the others (see below).

ENERGY STRUCTURE OF THE MARMAS

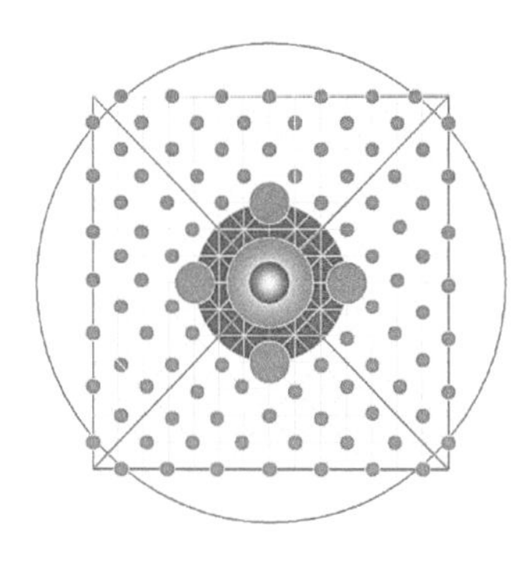

*A Marma includes minor points and acts as a coordination centre and switching point for energy pathways. Energetically, all 108 Marmas are represented. In the centre, the bindu, are the seven Mahamarmas.*

Since a Marma is more an area than a single point, it often includes several smaller Marmas and then acts as a coordinating centre, monitoring all the signals emanating from the smaller points. Also, several meridians (called *Nadis* in Ayurveda) always merge within a main Marma, which acts as a reservoir of energy. In India the confluence of rivers is called *Sangam*. Although this is not a traditional term in Marma Therapy, we would like to introduce it here, because it describes precisely the importance and function of these superior Marmas.

Korean hand acupuncture indicates how many points and Nadis can be found just in the hands. It describes a large number of small vital points on the hand along micro meridians, and treats them in accordance with their connections to the organs (see below). The 'heart of the hand' Marma in the middle of the palm interlinks all these points and meridians and coordinates them. Several points and meridians also gather in the wrist Marma, *Manibandha*, and they are coordinated and controlled by that Marma.

SCHEMATIC REPRESENTATION OF KOREAN HAND ACUPUNCTURE POINTS

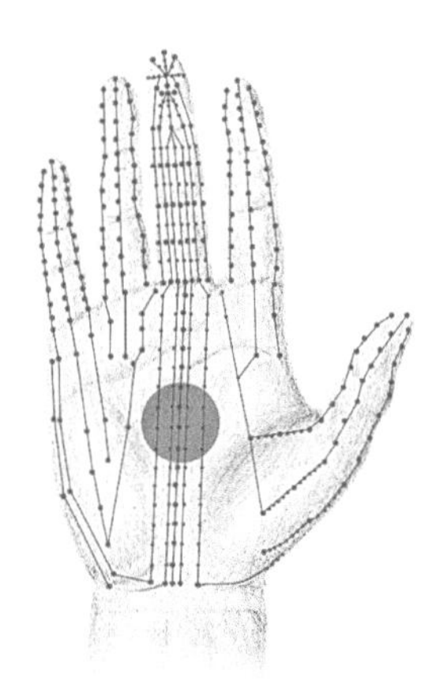

*Numerous vital points are connected by micro-meridians. Talahridaya acts as a coordination centre. (Image freely adapted from Dr. Yoo Tae Woo.)*

## The Marma house

A Marma is like a house in which all the residents have their own rooms and tasks. Here again we find all the Ayurvedic principles: the three Doshas as bioregulators, the five elements as components of the Marmas, the metabolic energy Agni, the happiness and nutrient substance Ojas, the seven types of tissue Dhatus, and the mental characteristics (*Sattva*, *Rajas* and *Tamas*). They all indicate the individual field of activity and significance of a Marma, and on this basis we can make a meaningful classification of the Marmas that will be useful in our treatment.

ALL ASPECTS ARE UNITED IN EACH MARMA

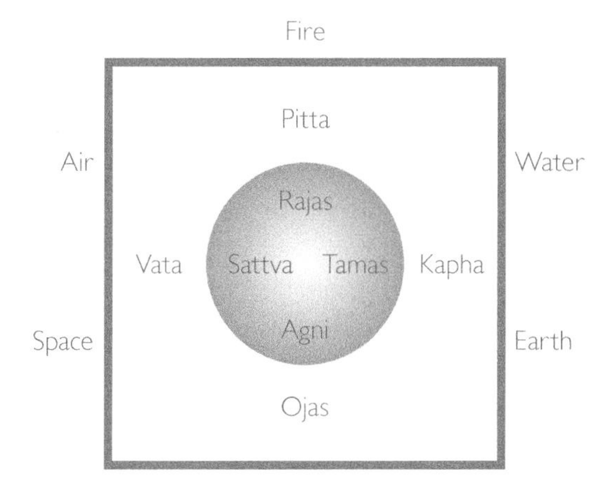


*All the Ayurvedic principles are present and operate in each Marma.*

### The three Doshas as bioregulators

The three Doshas characterize the function of a Marma. In some, Vata is predominant, for example in Marmas located in the joints. Their job is to control and coordinate motion and orientation in space. Marmas ruled by Pitta are responsible for metabolism and the generation of energy and heat. Kapha Marmas provide stability and endurance, and maintain the physical structure.

### The five elements as components of the Marmas

All five elements are generally represented in each Marma, but one or two may predominate, depending on the type of Marma. *Fire Marmas* warm or heat up. When treating them we feel a sensation of heat or warmth that even spreads along the corresponding energy channel. But there are also cooling Marmas where *water* is the dominant element. When the element of *air* or *space* dominates in a Marma, then it is particularly sensitive and alert and controls movement, as in the joint Marmas. Where the *earth* element predominates, the Marmas provide stability.

### Tissue types in Marma

Ayurveda divides body tissue into seven basic structure patterns. Some have more effect on plasma and lymph, others on blood, muscle, adipose tissue, bone and the supporting tissues of the body. They can also have a special reference to the brain or the reproductive organs.

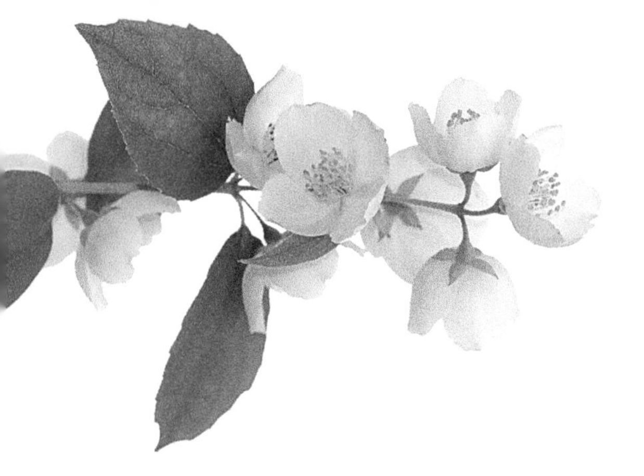

## Agni – the flame of life in Marma

Light and energy (Agni) are present in each Marma. Agni is the fire of life that underlies animate and inanimate nature as the principle of energy and heat. It is responsible for energy transformation and maturation, even in the mental sense. In the body we find Agni most obviously as the digestive fire. It 'burns' in the digestive organs, in all cells and anywhere where materials are processed and converted – and hence also in the Marmas.

## Ojas – the basis for happiness and nourishment in Marma

Ojas is the 'unifying substance' between mind and body in Marma. It too is like light, shining from consciousness into the body and from the body into consciousness. Furthermore Ojas is the basis for happiness, the best and most natural antidepressant. Ojas underlies the body's tissues and nourishes and organizes them.

## The three mental qualities

Ayurveda describes three mental qualities that shape the human personality and also characterize the Marmas. These are the three *Gunas* – Sattva, Rajas and Tamas. Sattva Marmas are of special spiritual significance. They reflect and support a pure mind and heart and serve for the realization of spiritual goals (for example, the major heart Marma or the supreme ruler Adhipati). Rajas Marmas energize and ignite passion (for example, the groin and pubic bone Marmas Lohitaksha and Vitapa). Tamas Marmas are the conservative ministers in the state. They want to preserve, maintain and also restrain, are more insensitive and materialistic, and often act like shields (for example, the shoulder blade Marma Amsaphalaka).

## Ama – toxins in Marma

Ama is the opposite of Ojas and refers to impurities in the body and mind. Literally, '*A-ma*' means 'not digested'. Everything we have not digested mentally and physically acts as Ama, as well as the toxins we ingest from outside the body, such as environmental toxins, some drugs or contaminated food. Ama can accumulate in the Nadis and block the flow of energy or it can sit in the Marmas and make them dull, impairing their perception and awareness and generating irritation or malfunction in these physical control centres.

Traditionally, Marmas are also distinguished by two further criteria: the consequences of injury and the predominant tissue type.

## Classification of Marmas by the consequences of injury

Traditionally, Marmas are classified according to the consequences of injury. Indeed, the medical knowledge of Marmas is based on the ancient Indian martial art Kalari, which is still practised today in South India. In Kerala, young men are taught the traditional *Kalari Payat*, where they learn discipline, control of the body, mental concentration and how to establish the integrated state of unity consciousness within themselves. In the adjacent state of Tamil Nadu, at the southernmost tip of the Indian subcontinent, this traditional Vedic martial art is called *Kalari Payirchi*.

At first glance, these different reactions to injury do not appear to be so important – at least in peacetime. But the type of reaction following an injury actually gives important information about the likely response of a Marma to a healing treatment and its sensitivity to that treatment.

MARMAS AND THE CONSEQUENCES OF INJURY

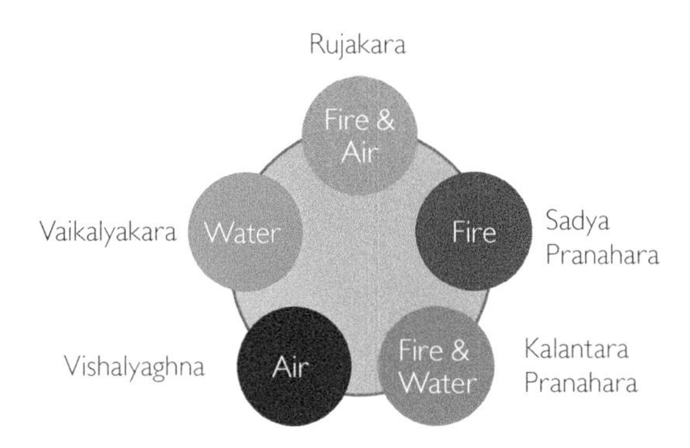


*The five elements determine the energetic quality and the type of reaction of the Marmas.*

Actually, it is the five elements that are responsible for these different reactions: Marmas which are dominated by fire react strongly to injuries; air Marmas are very sensitive to pain; and water Marmas react slowly, with a disturbance causing weakness.

This knowledge has potential significance for modern surgery: a section through a Marma can act as an interference field and can cause lasting complaints or recurring blockages.

## Differences between Marmas according to the predominant tissue type

A Marma area is defined as a place where five types of tissue meet: muscle, blood vessels, tendons, bones and joints. Sometimes nerves are also mentioned. At every point one of these tissue elements dominates. Thus, we can distinguish 11 muscle, 41 blood vessel, 27 tendon, 8 bone and 20 joint Marmas (see chart on page 22).

## Types of Marma

**Mamsa – Muscle**

- Stanarohita (2×)
- Indrabasti (4×)
- Talahridaya (4×)
- **Guda** (1×)

*Promote power, strengthen Agni, store energy, centrally located.*

*Have predominantly Kapha–Pitta qualities.*

**Sira – Vessels**

- Apanga (2×)
- **Sthapani** (1×)
- Shringataka (4×)
- Phana (2×)
- Sira Matrika (8×)
- **Manya** (2×)
- **Nila** (2×)
- Apalapa (2×)
- Lohitaksha (4×)
- Apastambha (2×)
- Stanamula (2×)
- Brihati (2×)
- **Hridaya** (1×)
- **Nabhi** (1×)
- Parshvasandhi (2×)
- Urvi (2×)
- Bahvi (2×)

*Control the blood supply, blood flow and temperature homeostasis.*

*Have predominantly Pitta qualities.*

**Asthi – Bone**

- Shankha (2×)
- Amsaphalaka (2×)
- Nitamba (2×)
- Katikataruna (2×)

*Protect the sensitive and pain-sensitive areas of the body, provide stability.*

*Have predominantly Vata–Kapha qualities.*

**Sandhi – Joint**

- **Adhipati** (1×)
- Simanta (5×)
- Avarta (2×)
- Krikatika (2×)
- Kurpara (2×)
- Manibandha (2×)
- Kukundara (2×)
- Janu (2×)
- Gulpha (2×)

*Are the sensors in the joint, coordinate stability, dance, movement, sensitivity, susceptible to Vata and spatial orientation.*

*Have predominantly Vata and Shlesha-ka–Kapha qualities.*

**Snayu – Tendon**

- Vidhura (2×)
- Utkshepa (2×)
- Kakshadhara (2×)
- Amsa (2×)
- Ani (4×)
- **Basti** (1×)
- Vitapa (2×)
- Kurchashira (4×)
- Kurcha (4×)
- Kshipra (4×)

*Express elasticity, speed, adaptability and strength.*

*Have predominantly Vata–Kapha qualities.*

The figure shows an overview of all 107 Marmas as they are classified traditionally by the type of tissue they control and in which they are predominantly located. The seven Mahamarmas are shown in bold type (Nila–Manya together are considered as one of the seven central Marmas).

# Types of Marma Therapy

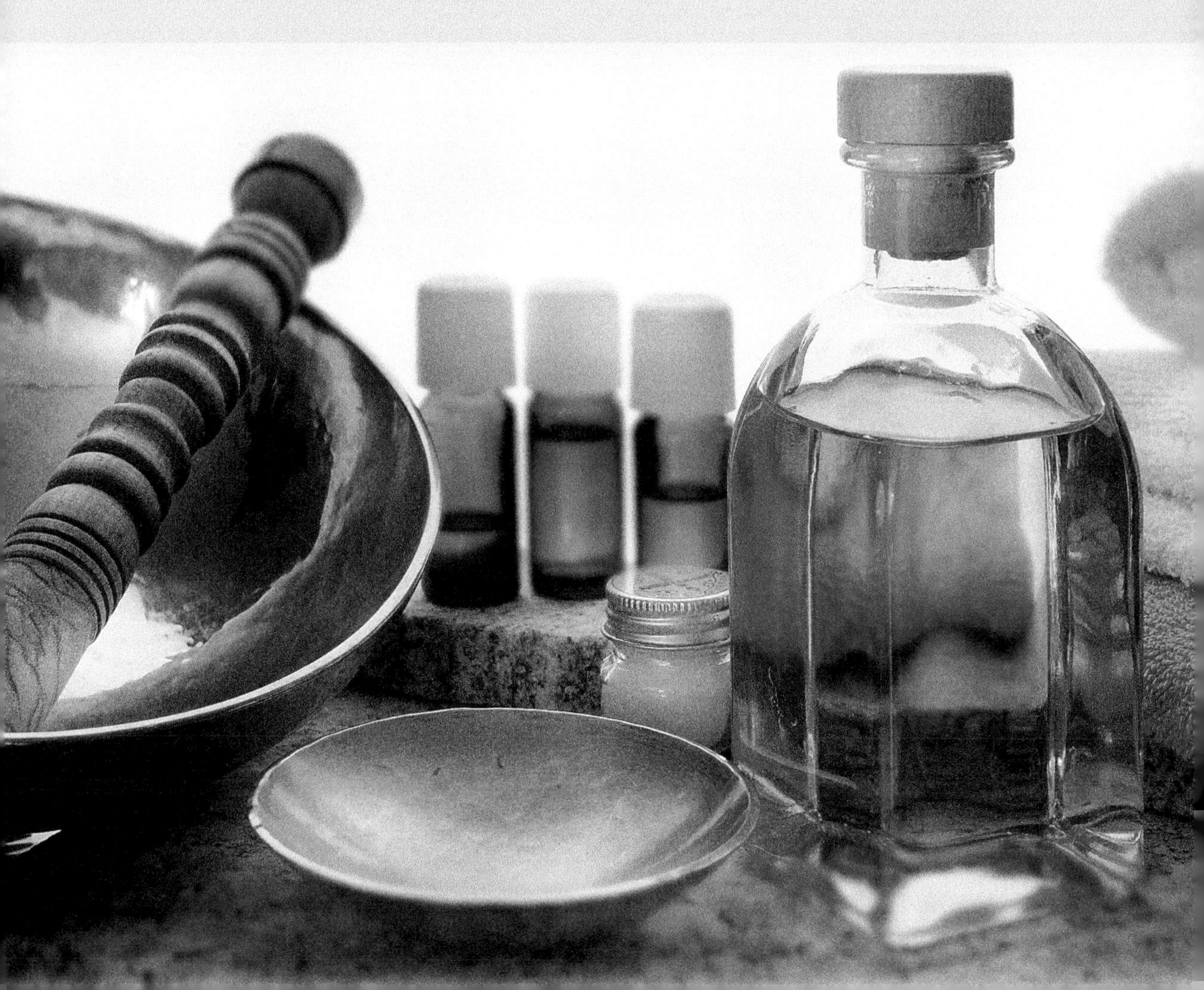

# Different Treatment Methods

Marma points can be treated in very different ways. Massage with and without oil is the usual way. But even directing attention to a Marma without touching it has a strong and distinct effect. To feel this, sit comfortably but upright, close your eyes and take a deep breath calmly through the nose, in and out. Then direct your attention to a Marma. It can be a relatively small one such as *Kshipra*, the Marma between the thumb and forefinger, or a big one like the heart or bladder Marma. If you feel into it very naturally, you will enliven it. You feel its energy, perhaps even the feelings stored in it, or part of its function. Sometimes it is even possible to follow the course of a meridian which comes to or from the Marma.

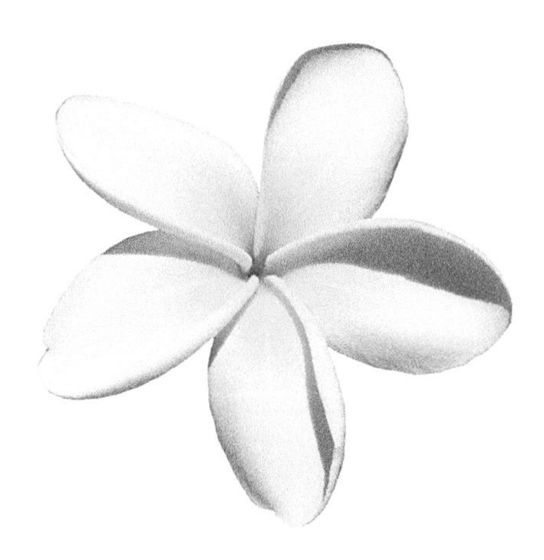

## 20 WAYS TO TREAT MARMAS

1. Pure attention without touching
2. Touching with attention
3. Marma massage with or without oil
4. Oil bath on a Marma: Basti
5. Ointment on a Marma: Ahajana
6. Pouring oil, ghee, lassi or other liquids onto the Marma: Marmadhara
7. Application with paste or herbal pulp: Lepam
8. Local application of heat, red light, hot stone therapy
9. Gem light therapy and colour therapy
10. Singing bowls
11. Herbal and mineral supplements: Rasayanas
12. Food, herbal teas, medicinal waters containing specific herbs and minerals
13. Metals, rings, jewellery
14. Aromatherapy
15. Vedic music and sound therapies: Gandharva-Veda, recitation of Vedic texts
16. Vedic ceremonies to strengthen positive influences: Yagya
17. Yoga exercises: Asanas
18. Finger and body positions: Mudras
19. Breathing exercises: Pranayama
20. Contemplation and meditation

## Proper touch heals

Mental contact is certainly the subtlest form of Marma Therapy. But, with its refinement and subtlety, simple touch with the hand comes very close. In daily life we often unconsciously touch certain Marmas. For example, when we have abdominal pain, we instinctively put our hand on the abdomen, with the palm just above the navel. In this way we soothe and strengthen the navel Marma, *Nabhi*, the ruler of the stomach and its organs. When we have a headache we touch or rub our temples, thus freeing the blocked flow in *Shankha*, the temple Marma. Also a mother often treats the Marmas of her child: if the child cries she strokes the head in a loving and consoling way, where *Adhipati*, the crown Marma, resides. Of all the Marmas, Adhipati has the most soothing influence on an aroused nervous system.

## Applying ointments, herbs and oils to a Marma point

Even in Western naturopathic medicine there are very well-known Marma applications, such as ointments, hot packs or herbal packs. Think about chest ointment for a cold. It opens the airways, supports the expectoration of mucus and has a liberating effect on bronchi and lungs. We rub the ointment exactly on the heart Marma, *Hridaya*, which is the energy centre for the entire chest region with all its organs. Ayurveda often uses sophisticated oils that are applied to the Marmas. (For example, the treatment known as *Shirodhara* involves pouring warm oil onto the forehead; while *Takradhara* uses cooling buttermilk or ghee.) There are other simple but effective treatments that can be used at home. If you are suffering from insomnia, anxiety or nervousness, take some drops of a soothing herbal oil and, in the evening before bedtime, rub it with the palm of your hand gently in a soothing manner on the top of your head. This is the area of Adhipati Marma, and this technique will promote peace, sleep and steady nerves.

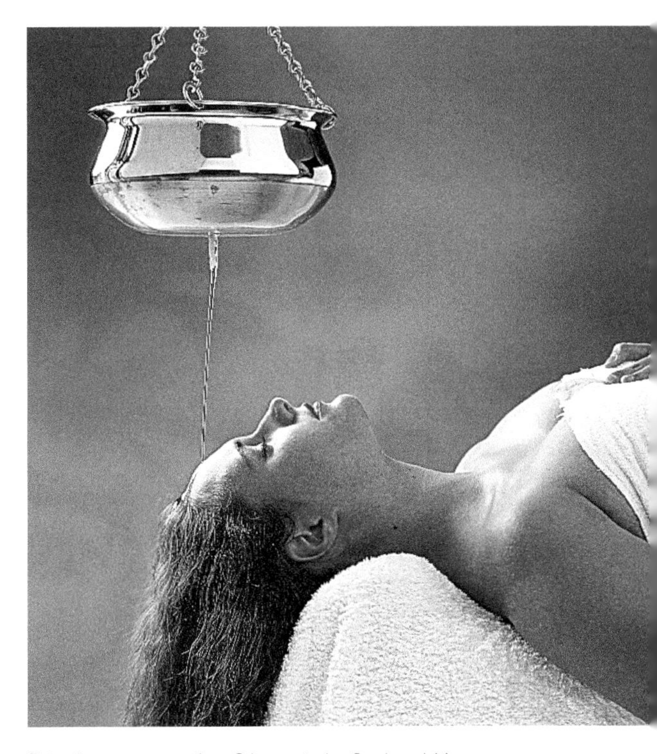

*Shirodhara: warm oil on Sthapani, the forehead Marma*

## Rasayanas – rejuvenation remedies of Ayurveda

Ayurveda is concerned with the preservation of youth and health. An important preventive therapeutic approach is the use of Rasayanas, plant and mineral supplements that nourish body and mind with the finest life-promoting nutrients. These sometimes lavishly manufactured preparations serve to transport the sap of life, *Rasa*, to all cells and organs so that the organizing intelligence of the physiology and wakeful awareness are maintained in the organism. In this way, Rasayanas always have a precise effect on the Marmas and Nadis, purifying them and keeping them functioning correctly. Of particular importance is their rejuvenating influence on the major fields of consciousness in the body, the Mahamarmas. For example, the fruit of the Amla tree, which grows widely throughout India, clears the third eye, *Sthapani*, and strengthens Ojas in the heart and navel Marmas. The *Brahmi* plant is a precious nerve and brain medicine that promotes memory and concentration and acts specifically on the crown Marma *Adhipati*. Long pepper (Sanskrit: Pippali) is one of the best herbs to strengthen the digestive fire. It has a strong purifying influence on the transportation channels of the body, and also on the energy pathways and Marmas in general. Pippali primarily strengthens the navel Marma, but also the two eye Marmas *Avarta* and *Apanga*. In the chapter 'Marma Therapy for Everyday Complaints' (page 127) we will come back to the Rasayanas and discuss specific applications.

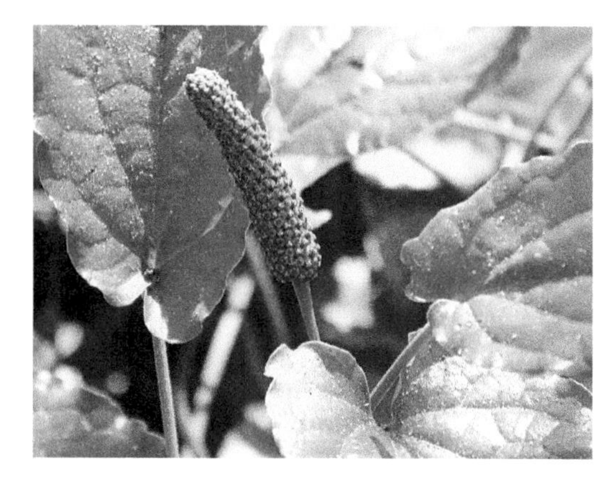

*Long pepper – leaves and fruit*

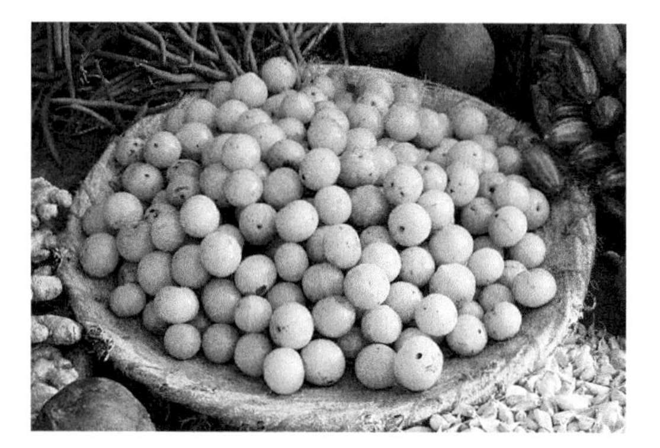

*Amla fruit*

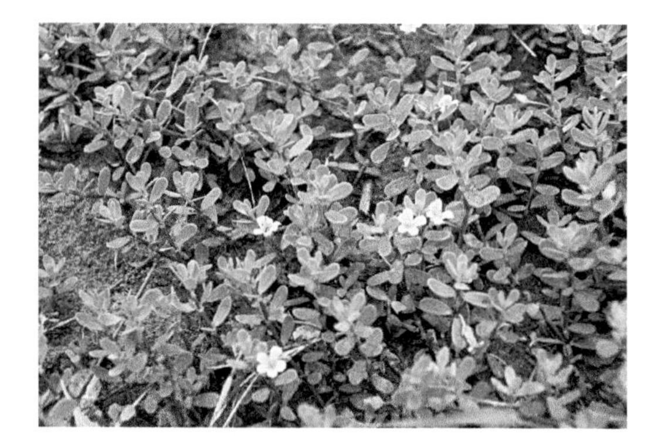

*Brahmi – plant with flowers*

## Oil bath on a Marma

There is another Ayurvedic treatment where oils are applied directly on a Marma, which has a profound effect. This therapy is called a local *Basti* – literally an enema. Basti in Ayurveda has several meanings: the bladder, the bladder Marma, an enema or just an oil bath on a specific part of the body. The figure opposite shows *Kati Basti*, an oil bath on the Marmas of the lower back. An oil-impermeable ring made from a dough of flour and water is formed around this area. Then a warm medicinal herbal oil is poured in and left there for 20 minutes. During this time, the oil and medicinal plants have an extremely soothing and healing effect on all layers of the body: in the layer of consciousness of the aura above the skin, on the skin itself with its connections to internal organs, and in the inner organs up to the deeper layers and the muscles. *Kati Basti* mainly treats the Marmas of the sacroiliac joint, both the *Kukundaras* and also different, smaller vital points in the centre and on both sides of the spine. All the points get harmonized and energized with the healing essences, and the discord, the dissonant vibration that dominates in a disease, is absorbed and neutralized by the oil.

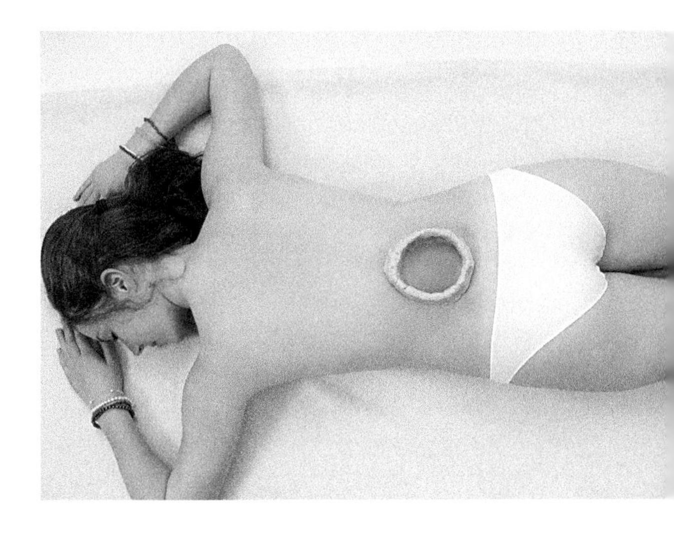

*Kati Basti – oil bath on lower back Marmas*

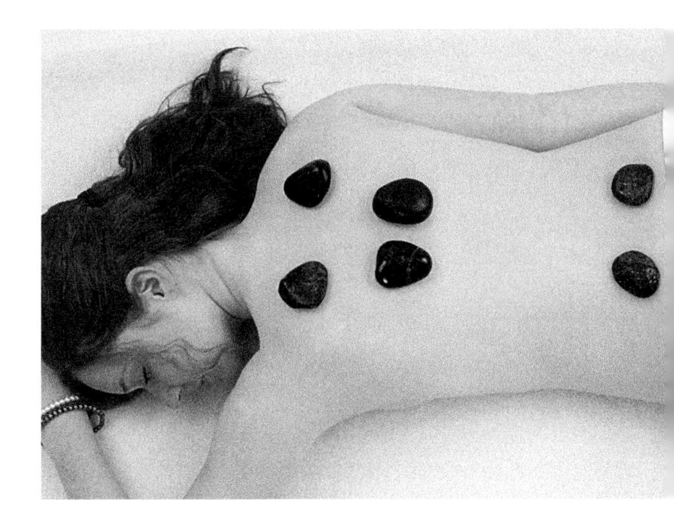

*Hot stone therapy can be used directly on the Marmas*

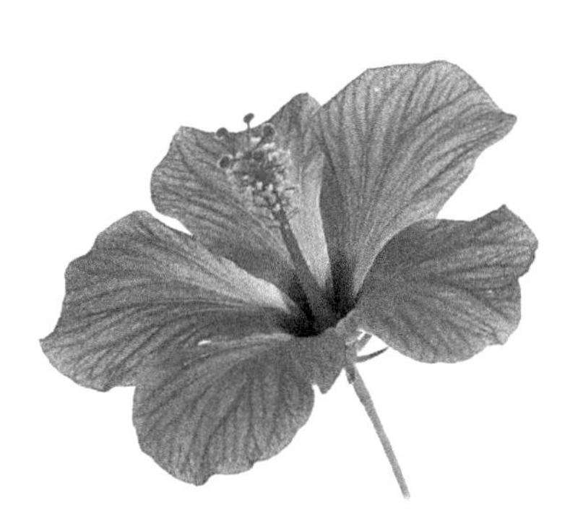

## Treatment through the five senses

Our senses are the gateways to our consciousness, which links all the Marmas. Every sensory perception – whether sight, smell, taste, sound or touch – acts directly on the Marmas. When we see red – or red light falls on our skin – then Pitta is stimulated in the Marmas. Blue, on the other hand, cools Pitta but increases Vata. Green calms over-stimulated Vata but strengthens Kapha. In the same way, blends of these three basic colours influence the system of the Doshas and Marmas. Marma Therapy can also utilize various spectra of light and healing energies provided by gemstones. We can put them directly on a Marma point, wear a ring on the appropriate finger, or radiate the Marmas with light projected through gemstones.

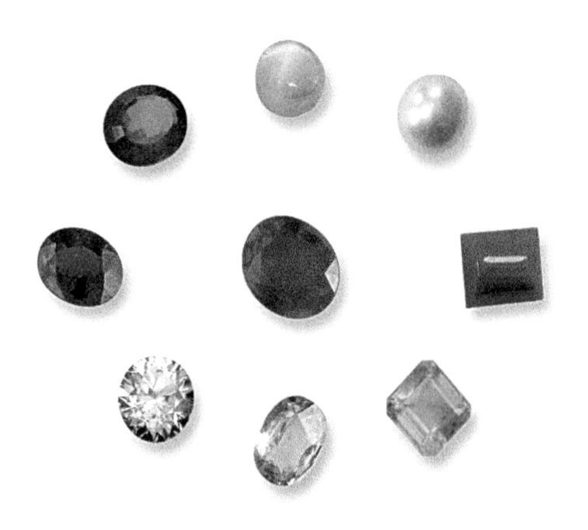

*Navaratna, the nine major gems used in Ayurvedic medicine*

Our mind–body system reacts to every sensory stimulus with its Marmas. The conscious use of a special taste in tea such as bitter, sweet or pungent, the calming fragrance of lavender, specific melodies, the frequencies of sound bowls or the sounds of nature resonate with the Marmas and harmonize them. Sound bowls can be used directly on the skin or over a Marma even without touching it.

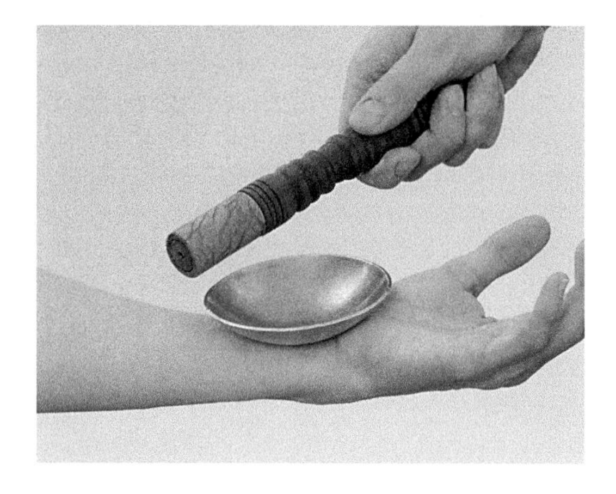

*Treatment of wrist Marmas with a singing bowl*

## Marmas respond to sound and music

Marmas are like highly sensitive broadcasting and receiving stations sharing information between the inner nature of man and the frequencies of the environment. Any change in consciousness affecting our vibration generates direct effects on the information content and the vibration of Marma points.

An extraordinary experiment illustrates this (see below). If you measure the skin resistance of the small Marma or acupuncture points on the fingers or toes and represent them graphically, then everyone has an individual graph, a kind of fingerprint of the energy charge in these Marmas (see below right). This provides a description of energetic balance, of health and illness. In the experiment, the subject's initial measurement curve is narrow (blue line), the energy of the vital points is weak, and the loop is not circular, showing imbalance. When the subject listened to Vedic sounds (a recitation of Rig Veda) for a few minutes, the picture improved extraordinarily. The circle of measurement points is significantly wider, energy levels have increased and the measurement curve is now nearly perfectly circular. This means that the Marmas being measured have become very balanced energetically, which is a sign of great harmony in the physiology.

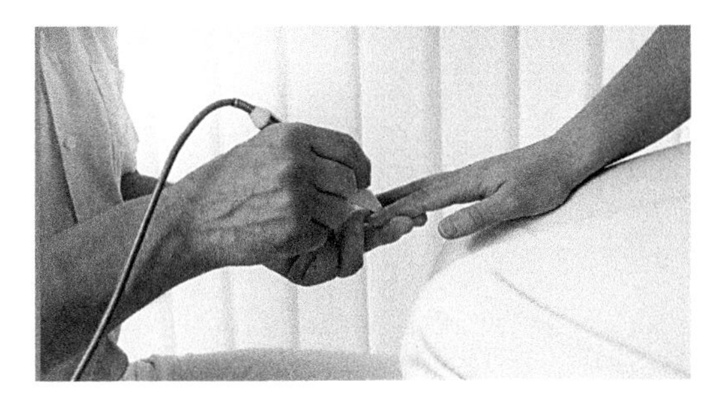

*Measurement of skin resistance at Marma points*

Vedic music therapy, Gandharva Veda, is particularly easy to utilize. It is composed according to diurnal rhythms and there are recordings of gentle melodies and sounds for each hour of the day. Whether instrumental or vocal, this music calms the mind in minutes and directly leads it within, back to the source of all Marmas, to the Self. Even five to ten minutes' listening to this healing music is sufficient to harmonize the Marmas effectively and noticeably.

THE EFFECT OF VEDIC RECITATION ON THE ENERGY LEVEL OF MARMA POINTS

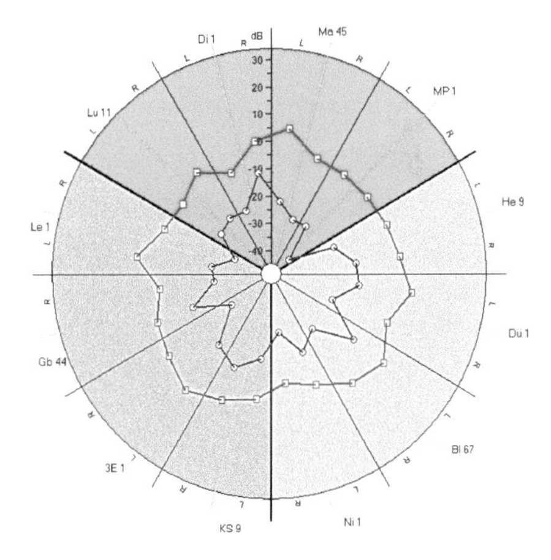


*Measurement curve of skin resistance of Marma points. Blue curve = before, red curve = six minutes after listening to Rig Veda recitation. The line forms an almost perfect circle, falling within the optimal range for skin resistance.*

## Marmas and meditation

Meditation is a very effective mental technique to harmonize the various Marmas in our body, to charge them with Prana, life energy, and to strengthen and restore order and health in mind and body. Transcendental Meditation, which comes directly from the Vedic tradition, uses a sound, a *mantra*, which leads the mind effortlessly and without concentration from the dense levels of thinking to silence without thought. In this context, the mantra is not merely a convenient vehicle for the mind, it also has a direct healing effect on the Marmas in the body.

## Yoga, Mudras and breathing exercises

Physical Yoga exercises, *Asanas*, give the Marmas room to breathe. They reconnect the Marmas with the state of unity, the inner Self, the Atma. When they are reconnected in this way, the Marmas are enlivened, they expand and can fully express their inner qualities. The heart Marma, Hridaya, for example, can then express more love, more emotional intelligence and more holistic values.

Yoga Asanas charge the Marmas with energy and support physical and mental reprocessing of the patterns of experience stored in the Marmas. In addition, certain finger postures, or *Mudras*, can be used to harmonize the Marmas. Two short chapters are specifically devoted to Mudras and Asanas (page 110 and page 119). We also describe some simple breathing exercises that can be used to strengthen and harmonize Prana and thus bring energy to the Marmas and Nadis.

## The Yagya ceremony

In the Ayurvedic approach to health a ceremony that addresses the Divine in creation and brings our consciousness in touch with it is called a *Yagya*. A Yagya is a ceremonial act, traditionally practised by Vedic *Pandits*. It creates a healing, protecting and blessing influence for the person for whom it is performed. In fact, any prayer, every good thought or meditation that brings us back to the silence of the heart could be described as a Yagya. The same applies to a good life in harmony with yourself and the laws of nature or the ritual of a priest in front of an altar. According to Vedic teaching, each Marma represents a divine principle of action, a law of nature, *Devata*. Marmas which have been charged with negative emotions and patterns of experience can be healed through the principle of Yagya.

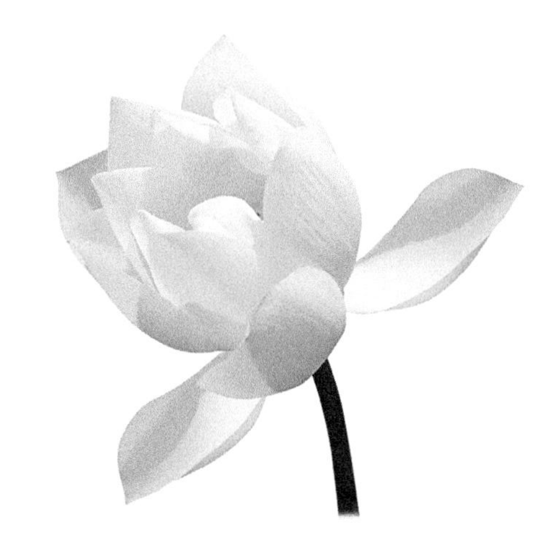

# Treatment Techniques

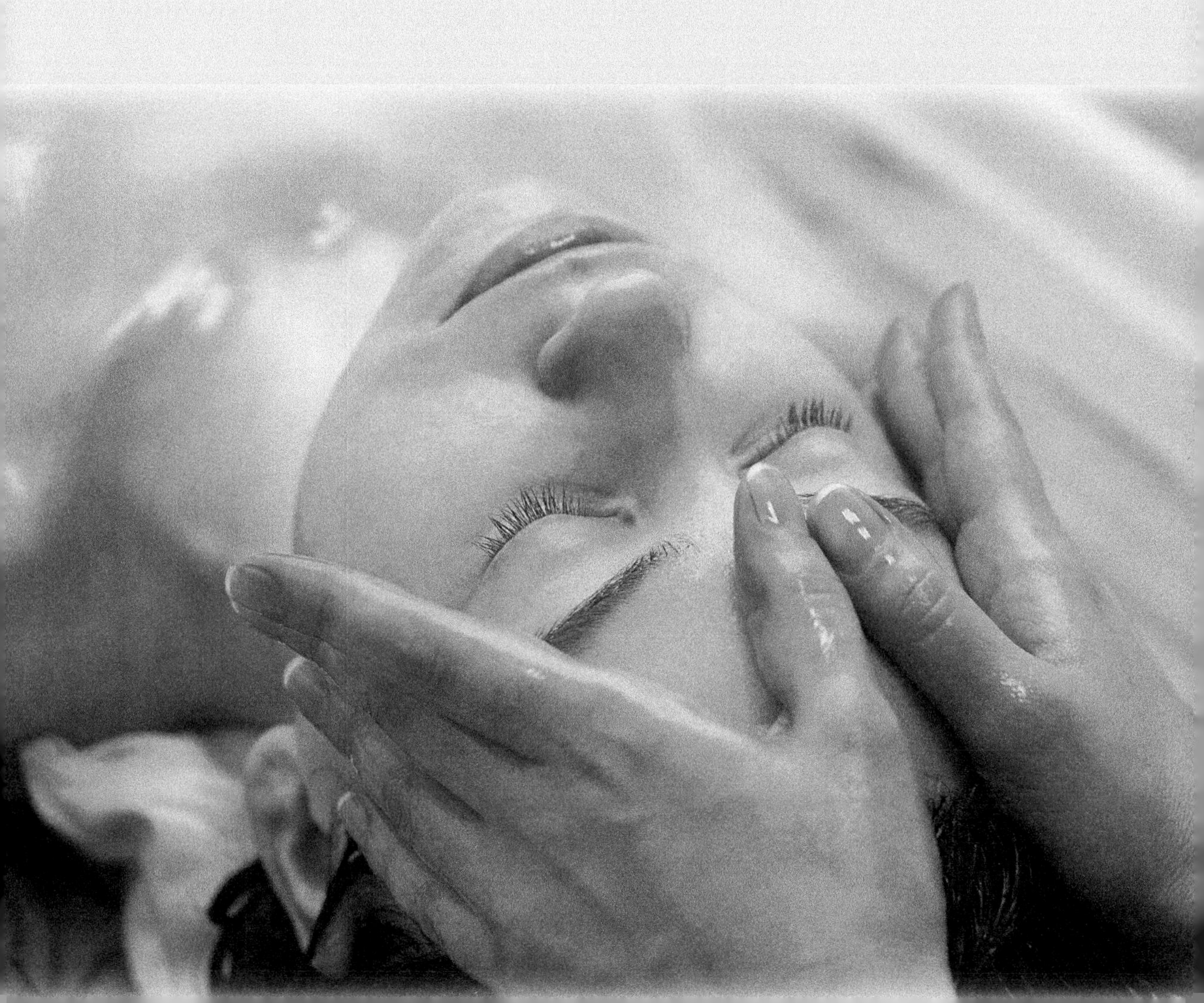

# General Rules for Marma Treatment

Only when it is simple and very natural can Marma Therapy be at its most effective. All the various techniques – the influence of individual fingers of the treating hand, the selection of the correct oil, the choice and sequence of the points to treat – extend the possibilities and improve the effect. But nothing is as important as you yourself, your attitude, your attention and calmness during the treatment and the naturalness of how you touch, feel and treat the Marmas. Your fingers should naturally flow and glide and you should always approach a treatment with the intention of generating well-being.

## Preparing for a treatment

Before you begin, settle down for a moment. Close your eyes, breathe in and out deeply and collect yourself until your thoughts settle down. At the start of treatment, you (or your partner) can do pranayama (page 126) for two or three minutes. This subtle breathing technique is soothing, has been scientifically proven to harmonize left and right hemispheres and gives healing energy, Prana, to the Marmas and Nadis.

## The importance of pressure in massage

Marmas and Nadis can be treated more on a physical level or more on the level of consciousness. In the West, the traditional massage technique for connective tissue or the muscles generally involves strong pressure. Similarly, Marma massage in South India, especially in Siddha medicine, is usually performed with distinct, sometimes very strong and even painful pressure and with rapid movements. This can help to dissolve swelling in the tissues, reduce stiffness in muscles or release blockages. However, if you experience a very gentle treatment with a good herbal oil, then you will notice a major difference between gentle and strong pressure: the gentle method acts on the level of consciousness where the Marmas have their origin, while the firmer technique acts mainly on the level of the body. The techniques that we describe in this book for self and partner treatment are almost all gentle and lead to inner peace. Therefore they act primarily on the level of consciousness and only secondarily on the body and its organs.

## The strokes

These different strokes and circular motions are key features of Sukshma Marma Therapy:

- **Circular massage on the Marma point:** A clockwise movement stimulates the Marma; counterclockwise calms it or has a detoxifying effect via the corresponding energy and physiological channels and organs.

- **Massage with longitudinal strokes:** Longitudinal strokes move energy along the Nadis and free the channel of energy blocks and deposits. Up-and-down strokes also activate the metabolism in the Nadi. Strokes in a particular direction either support the energy flow or calm it, according to the direction of the flow of energy in the Nadi.

- **The distributive massage:** Strokes sideward or downwards away from a Marma are often performed when the Marma has to be relieved, for example after an injury, or to distribute congested energy in the case of a disease.

- **Draining or energy-building massage:** Basic and draining massages are performed from the top downwards, for example from shoulder to hand. Energy-creating massages, however, run the other way round – upwards – for example from the sacrum to the top of the head when the Prana from the lower Marmas has to be brought to the crown Marma.

- **Vigorous rubbing:** Fast and powerful rubbing of a painful or tense area distributes congested energy and brings immediate relief.

- **Tapping or light clapping:** We can awaken a Marma with a dosed tapping on a Marma with the middle finger (which carries the qualities of Pitta). In this way Prana is stimulated and set in motion. For larger Marmas soft clapping with the palm of the hand has a similar effect. In the South Indian martial art of Kalari (see also page 21) the combatants enliven intense energy impulses by clapping themselves strongly on the thigh Marmas during a fight.

- **Touching without massage:** This method works amazingly well. Here, we just put the thumb, the fingers or hand peacefully and in a supportive way on the Marma. This can be done with or without oil.

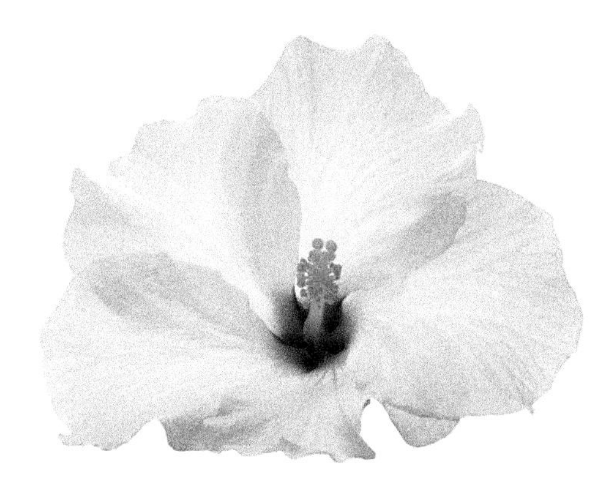

## The number of massage strokes – the 1–3–5–7 format

From our rational Western perspective it would seem that the number of consecutive circles or strokes in a treatment sequence can make no difference to the body. The Vedic sages, however, developed an understanding concerning which areas of human physiology are addressed by specific numbers of massage movements. For most Marmas we will keep to a certain sequence that we can call the *1–3–5–7 format*:

- **1** circle or up-and-down stroke on the Marma stimulates the formation of the finest fluid, Ojas, and starts its flow.
- **3** circles or stroking movements harmonize the three Doshas and bring them into tune.
- **5** circles or stroking movements in a row touch the five elements, *Mahabhutas*, and create balance in them.
- **7** circles or stroking movements transport Ojas to the seven tissues or structural principles, the Dhatus, and strengthen them.

After each cycle there is a short rest on the Marma, during which the body's intelligence is able to operate and heal.

### A TREATMENT SCHEME FOR ALL MARMAS

You can also apply the 1–3–5–7 treatment format in self or partner treatment of individual Marmas (page 41) unless another format is indicated. In addition to this format, feel free to treat according to your feeling – when the treatment is carried out correctly then it will bring a sense of well-being, not only to the partner but also to you. This is also the case in self-treatment.

Massage can also be firmer and faster. Kapha people in particular initially respond better to this type of approach. They are generally less sensitive and feel a stronger pressure to be more pleasant. Also the number of strokes and circles in the treatment can differ. Every situation is new and each person is different, so your treatments should be adapted to the different requirements. Feel free to try both methods: the format recommended and your own personal approach, guided by your feeling for the Marma's treatment requirement.

### Bringing the point to silence

The gentle Marma treatment is particularly effective if we guide the Marma from silence to dynamism and then back to silence. We put the hand or finger tenderly on the point where we have previously applied some oil. Then we do very smooth circular or linear motions, slowing down before ending in stillness on the Marma, letting the hand or finger rest there for one or two breaths. We repeat this procedure for the Marmas as many times as is indicated in the therapy section.

### Treat clockwise

Based on the right hand, all applications in this book are performed in a clockwise circular motion unless indicated otherwise. For the left hand, the movement is anti-clockwise.

Alternative procedures based on medical experience are applicable, but only in individual cases and therefore cannot be presented here.

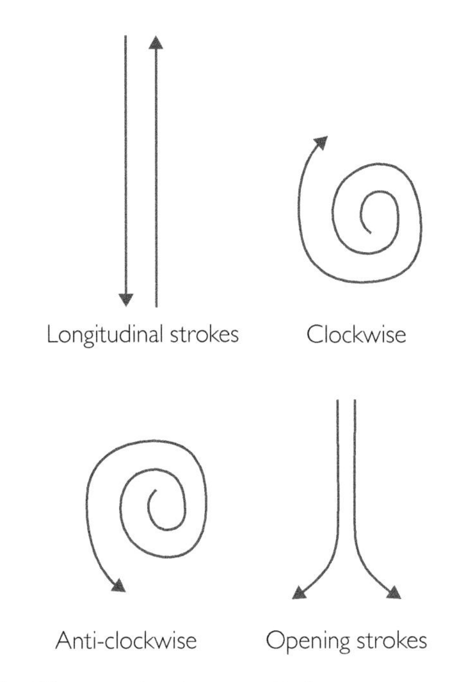


*The different strokes shown graphically*

## The significance and effects of fingers and the palm of the hand

Each finger has a special energetic aura and effect based on the five elements of Ayurvedic medicine, as follows:

- Thumb: space (and all the other elements)
- Index finger: air
- Middle finger: fire
- Ring finger: water
- Little finger: earth.

The *thumb* contains all properties, and its tip represents the central nervous system, the brain. From it flows Prana, life-energy. It is very well suited for treating small and medium Marmas. On the *index finger* we find *Vata*, on the *middle finger Pitta* and on the *ring finger Kapha*. With these fingers, we can systematically balance disturbed Doshas. So, for example, we can calm excessive Vata by using the Pitta or Kapha finger, or both together. Prana is also concentrated in *the centre of the palm*. *Talahridaya*, the heart of the hand, will therefore often be used in a treatment especially if we want to bring peace and strength to a Marma. This is often the best method when dealing with large Marmas.

### Which hand should we treat with?

According to Ayurveda, the right hand is under the influence of the sun, and from it warming energy emerges. The left hand is nurtured more by the moon, and has a more cooling effect. Generally we treat with the right hand whenever it is convenient and practical. The left one then supports on the other side of the treatment point. But there are areas of the body we can reach more easily with the left hand or with one of its fingers. In this case, the right hand will support. So take it easy: it is more important to feel comfortable rather than strain to follow a rule, since only with comfort are healing powers able to flow.

### Note for left-handers

For you it is the other way round. When the right hand is indicated, you treat with your dominant left hand and vice versa.

## Marmas inside and out – a harmonious partnership

All Marmas on the back and outer parts of the body have a more protective role. They tend to be less sensitive and have a male nature. The points on the inside and front of the body are more receptive and have perceptual properties. They are generally more sensitive and delicate and are of a female nature. The outer and inner points thus behave like a father and mother or a husband and wife in a perfect partnership or marriage, each offering support to the other in their own way.

▶ **The importance of the support point:** Each Marma has a support or counterpoint which lies exactly opposite it. For example, the supporting point of the central Marma in the palm, Talahridaya, can be found exactly opposite on the back of the hand. In classical Indian dance, even this outer Marma is painted (see page 110). The support Marma is extremely important in treatments. When we are massaging a Marma with one hand, we place the other protectively on its counter-point. Marmas are fields of consciousness in the body; they are tender, sensitive and vulnerable. If we protect the Marma, it feels safe and can open up confidently with all its potential to our therapy.

## Choosing the right oil

The correct choice of oil is extremely important because a good part of the healing effect of a Marma treatment comes from the plant ingredients and aromatic substances that the Marma receives. We can use high quality ready-made oils and blends or we can mix our own Marma oil. First you will need a body-friendly base oil which is suitable for massage. You may already have an oil for your treatments. It will be more effective if you add a few drops of a specially chosen essential oil. The feature on the far right gives you some hints.

▶ In **Vata disorders** or for very sensitive Vata-dominated people, base oils such as sweet almond, sesame or jojoba are very suitable.

▶ **Pitta** on the other hand feels more comfortable with coconut oil, sunflower oil or ghee. These have a cooling quality and balance excess Pitta. The sun-sensitive, light, often freckled skin of Pitta personalities tolerates these oils better. You can also use and apply clarified butter (ghee) directly on the Marma or, as discussed later in the book, mix it with another substance into a paste and then apply or rub it in.

▶ The more oily **Kapha skin** or a general Kapha accumulation in the individual requires oils that stimulate the metabolism such as sesame oil, to which you may add a stimulating, invigorating and thus Kapha-reducing essential oil.

Aroma oils are available in specialist shops (see page 141) but look out for purity and quality. The high-quality *VedAroma-Oils®* of Maharishi Ayurveda and *Oshadhi* oils are especially suitable for this purpose and meet all requirements for an effective fragrance for Marma treatment. The information on the right shows oils that are easy to obtain and their suitability for different Doshas. The Adhimarma oils mentioned in the book are special Marma oils with a targeted but also balancing effect on the individual Marmas that have been created specially for Sukshma Marma Treatment. Adhimarma oils (and many of the other oils mentioned) are available in the UK from *Oshadhi* (oshadhi.co.uk).

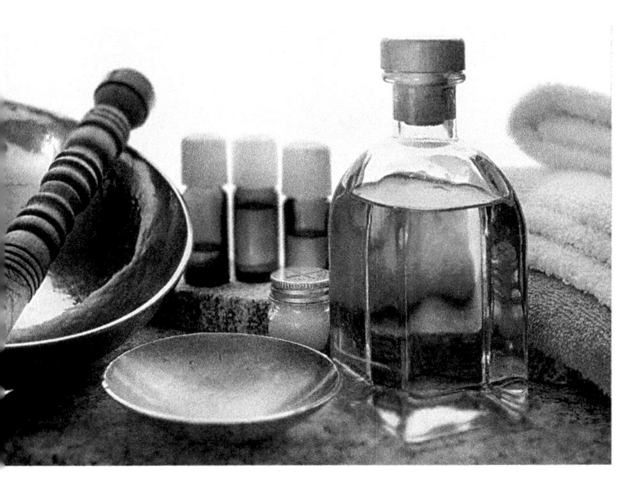

*Treatment utensils*

## Prepare the oils

Sesame oil should be 'ripened' before use, which means heating it briefly to boiling point. Ripened oils are also available in stores (see page 141). Before the treatment starts, warm the oil slightly and have it ready in a bowl, perhaps conveniently placed on a stool covered by a towel. Then add a few drops of an aromatic oil as needed into the oil base and mix it in. The Marma oil is ready.

## OILS FOR MARMA TREATMENT

### Vata-soothing (warming, antispasmodic, calming heavy oils)

Anise, cinnamon, cedar, calamus, clove (also pain relieving), frankincense (also anti-inflammatory), fennel (also antiflatulent), geranium, nutmeg (has a strong calming effect on the nervous system), valerian, jasmine (mentally uplifting), lemon, orange, lemongrass (also refreshing), rose (also for sorrow or heart ache), rosewood, basil, lotus (also spiritually uplifting), Brahmi (strengthens the nervous system), arnica and comfrey (both have pain-relieving qualities after injury)

**Base oils:** sweet almond, sesame, jojoba

**Finished products:** Vata massage oil, Heavenly Peace massage oil, Joint Soothe or MA 628 joint oil (pain, muscle and joint pain, arthritis)

**Aroma oils:** Nidra Aroma (for deep sleep), Smooth Cycle (for menstrual discomfort)

**Specific Marma oils (Adhimarma):** Shanti Om, Udana, Adhipati, Hridaya, Basti, Nidra Marma

### Pitta-balancing (cool, sweet-smelling oils)

Rose, sandalwood, mint (mainly cooling), coriander, camphor, chrysanthemum, lemongrass (also refreshing), myrrh, frankincense, vetiver

**Base oils:** coconut, ghee (clarified butter), sunflower

**Finished products:** Pitta massage oil

**Aroma oils:** Pitta aroma oil, MA 634 mint oil, Even Temper (emotional Pitta disorders)

**Adhimarma:** Hridaya, Indra Royal, Mahaojas

### Kapha-reducing (invigorating, light, bitter-tart, spicy-hot, opening or warming oils)

Ginger, clove, marjoram, ajowan, anise, rosemary, camphor, calamus, juniper, pine, eucalyptus

**Base oil:** sesame

**Finished products:** Kapha massage oil

**Aroma oils:** Kapha aroma oil, MA 634 mint oil (congestion; also for inhalation), Blissful Joy (depressive mood)

**Adhimarma:** Nabhi

## The order of treatment of individual Marmas

You may choose to treat a single Marma – the properties of, and treatment for, each Marma are described individually in the next chapter. However, it is more effective and of course part of the medical art to select a suitable combination of Marmas depending on the health disorder and to treat them in the right sequence. However, for this purpose extensive medical and Ayurvedic knowledge and skills are required, which is available on training courses in Marma Therapy but is beyond the scope of this book. However, we have indicated some standard protocols for everyday complaints (page 127), and these can be successfully applied by following the guidelines in this book.

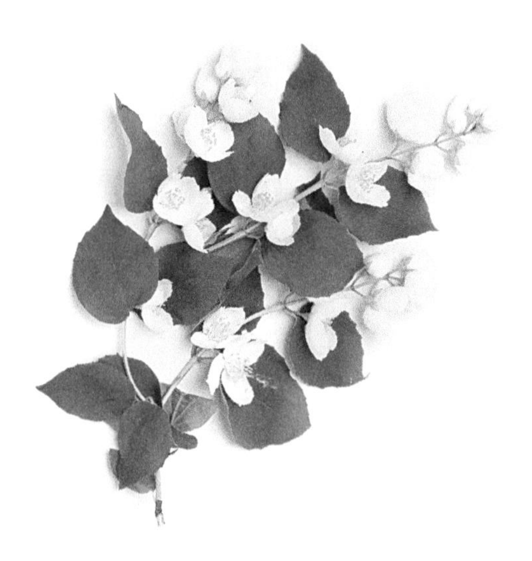

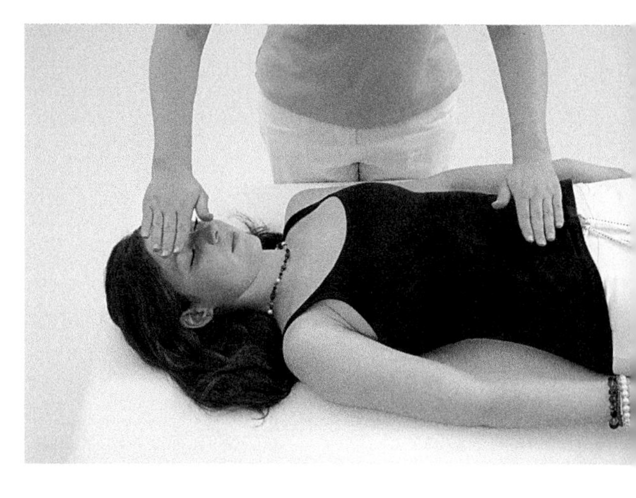

*Contact before a Marma treatment*

### Before treatment: making contact

We should start each major treatment by connecting with the three Mahamarmas of heart, bladder and forehead with our hands but without touching them physically. Our hands will rest a hand's breadth above the corresponding areas. Close your eyes and give these points attention for two or three breaths (see figure above). Start as shown in the photo, with the left hand over Basti and the right hand over Sthapani and, after a short while, move the left hand over Hridaya. This serves to attune ourselves with our partner, which we experience as a sense of well-being. We can also make direct contact with peripheral Marmas on the hands and feet by peacefully holding the Marmas for a few moments in our hands to give them a sense of security.

## Tips for self-treatment

There is a difference between treating yourself and treating somebody else. In self-treatment you can feel every Marma point precisely because it feels more sensitive. You also have a feeling for the right pressure, the number of circles required, the sense of well-being that comes during the treatment and possibly even for the effects on organs or other areas of the body that are connected to the treatment points.

### Important points for successful treatments

- Before you begin, prepare everything that you will need: a stool with a towel and a bowl with warm oil; a quiet room where you are able to relax and treat yourself undisturbed for a few minutes is ideal.

- Sit or lie comfortably. If you are sitting or lying on the floor, use a comfortable pad, a warm blanket or a Yoga mat.

- Breathe in and out once deeply and peacefully through the nose. This is relaxing and frees the mind of daily thoughts. Treat yourself sensitively with your eyes closed. Pay attention to the feedback from your body.

- The recommended number of circles and massage sequences is simply a guideline. Pay more attention to your well-being rather than internally counting and thus disturbing the actual treatment process.

- Relax for a few minutes after the treatment. Do not go immediately into the cold as the metabolism decreases during treatment. Stretch, move around and warm yourself up before going back to your activities.

- Enjoy your treatment, give yourself this valuable time and make this benefit for mind and body a regular procedure.

### ACCOMPANYING MUSIC?

Please, no background music! In this treatment you will lead the attention back into silence. Music, even if it is pleasant and relaxing, draws the attention outward while the treatment leads inwards – these are two opposite directions that would only create tension in the mind. However, you can listen to some relaxing music before treatment. The best results come from Maharishi Gandharva Music, which you can purchase in stores on CD or online (see page 141).

### Tips for partner treatment

Mindful attention is essential for the success of Marma Therapy! Partner treatment requires mindful attention and sensitivity in your hands. Ideally, you will feel how the energy of the other person starts to flow in the Marmas and Nadis as soon as you start the treatment. You may also notice that you will be guided by the consciousness of the other person. Their body's intelligence is particularly concentrated in the Marmas and this will guide you. You will become aware of how strong the pressure on a Marma needs to be during the massage and how slow or fast or how long the Marma point should be treated. During the whole treatment your partner should be relaxed and sit or lie quietly and he or she should have their eyes closed.

### Important information if you are treating another person

- Behave naturally and simply. Even if you are, do not act like a master or healer. Nature cures, you treat!

- Stay within yourself and in your silence. Breathe naturally and normally. Sit or stand comfortably during the treatment.

- Do not give energy intentionally! It is not about giving something, but about setting energy free. Even the simple touch of a Marma without any intention is itself a liberating impulse for healing or recovery.

- Marmas are the cosmic switchboards in our physiology and our role is to protect and strengthen and not to maltreat them. We should handle these vital points with care and sensitivity. This is of primary importance.

- Do not try to do more than nature allows or what is possible at that moment. Especially at the beginning, be satisfied with modest results. A little more well-being, a pleasant feeling of harmony in the patient and increased restfulness are the first signs of success. Often the effect is not present during the therapy itself but only afterwards. This is especially the case in specific bodily disorders.

- As laymen, do not treat diseases without consulting a physician.

### TREATMENT TIME

In the following section, the same treatment time applies to partner treatment as for self-treatment unless otherwise specified.

# Marmas: Meaning and Treatment

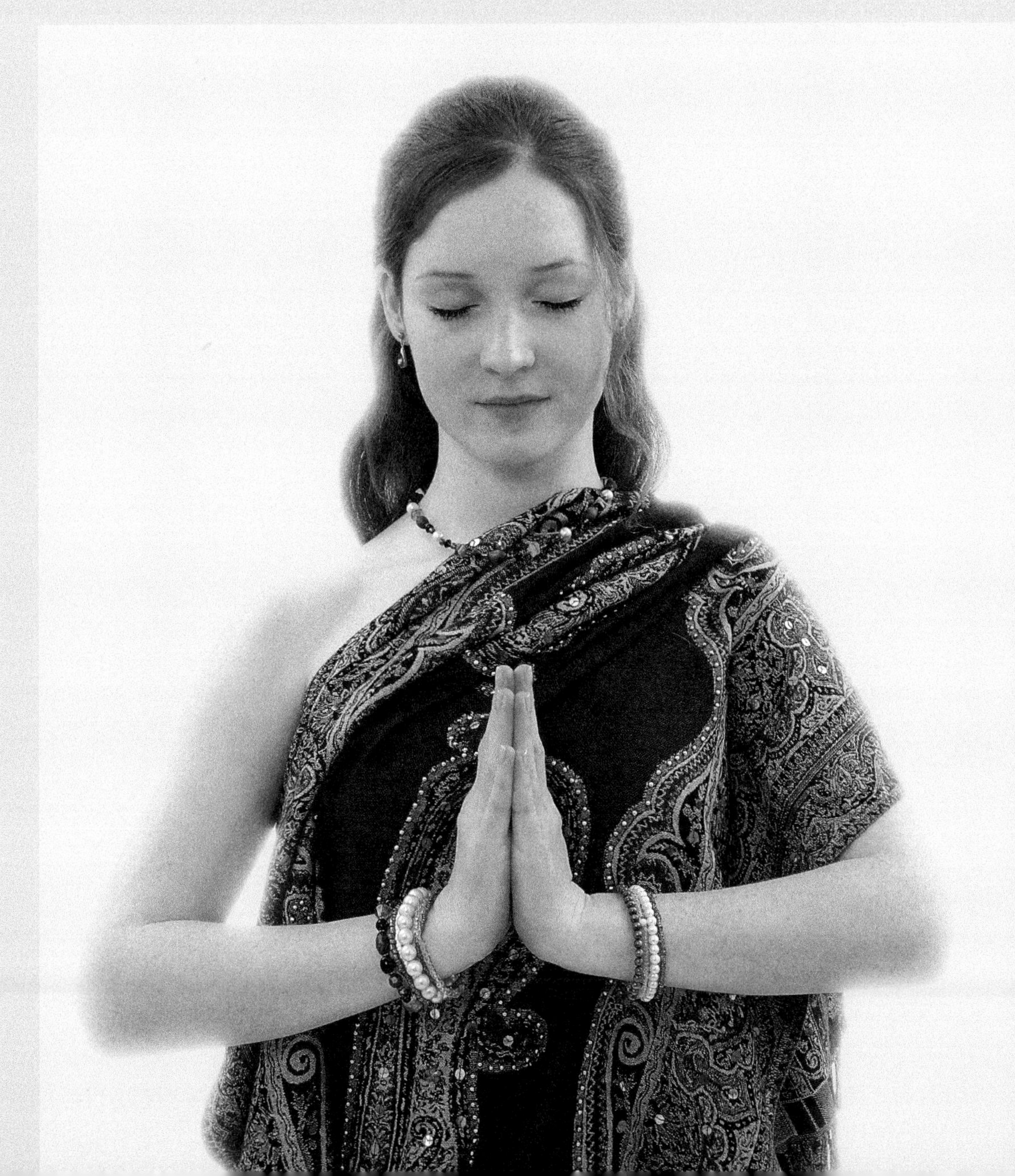

# Marmas on the Arms and Legs

The hands and feet are the peripheral representatives of the seven large Marmas which are located in the middle of the body. We can think of this 'central government' – with, as it were, its seven ministries – as having its 'outposts' on the hands and feet, and it is these that carry out the projects of the government and also report processes in the outer world to the central governmental ministries. This communication takes place via pathways in the arms and legs that function on a subtle energetic level. These are the Nadis connecting the Marmas. This communication is controlled and coordinated in special 'communication offices' which are the Marmas of the limbs.

On the hands there are a number of important Marmas that are mainly concerned with sensing, feeling, grasping and understanding the environment. These Marmas both give and receive. The Pranic energy is located with particular intensity on the fingertips and in the palm. The Marmas of the hand are therefore areas of concentrated healing power for treatment, touch and massage.

## THE PRANA OF THE WARRIORS

An ancient Vedic technology to vitalize Prana is to stretch the hands wide open to the sky, grasp the energy of the cosmos with the hands while breathing in deeply and then, during exhalation, pass the energy with the hands to specific Marmas on the body. This technique was mainly used by warriors in Vedic times in order to become charged with Prana and to strengthen and protect the Marmas.

While the hands are more controlled by the elements of air and space (making contact with the outside and up to the sky), the feet make contact with the ground and are the earthly counterpart, where the elements of earth and water dominate. (Note that in fact all elements and the three Doshas that are formed by them are present in all Marmas but with different dominances and to different degrees.) The arms and legs are traversed by numerous energy channels: Yoga scriptures describe two central Nadis (illustrated on page 43). They originate in Guda, the first of the seven Mahamarmas, flow through the bladder Marma – Basti – and are then distributed by the navel Marma into the arms and legs, which they provide with Pranic energy. These Nadis end in the centre of the palm and centre of the foot (Talahridaya Marma) from where the energy is distributed to the five fingers and toes and especially to the thumb and the big toe. The tips of the fingers and toes and especially the thumb and big toe are the openings of the Nadis to the outside and at the same time entry points for cosmic energy to be distributed to the Marmas of the hands and feet and to all other Marmas of the body.

The Marmas on the right side of the body and on the right arm and leg are of *solar* character and their treatment has a more warming effect, stimulating circulation and metabolism. It strengthens Agni (digestive fire) and increases Pitta. The Marmas on the left side of the body and on the left arm and leg are, on the other hand, of *lunar* quality, having a more cooling influence in treatments, reducing inflammation and supporting the development of body tissues, the Dhatus. They strengthen the functions dominated by Kapha or the water element in the body.

In addition to these central Nadis, there are at least six further important supply channels for the arms and legs, which Traditional Chinese Medicine (TCM) describes as meridians. The Marmas on the arms and legs are easily accessible for massage and other treatments and are therefore especially suited for self-treatment.

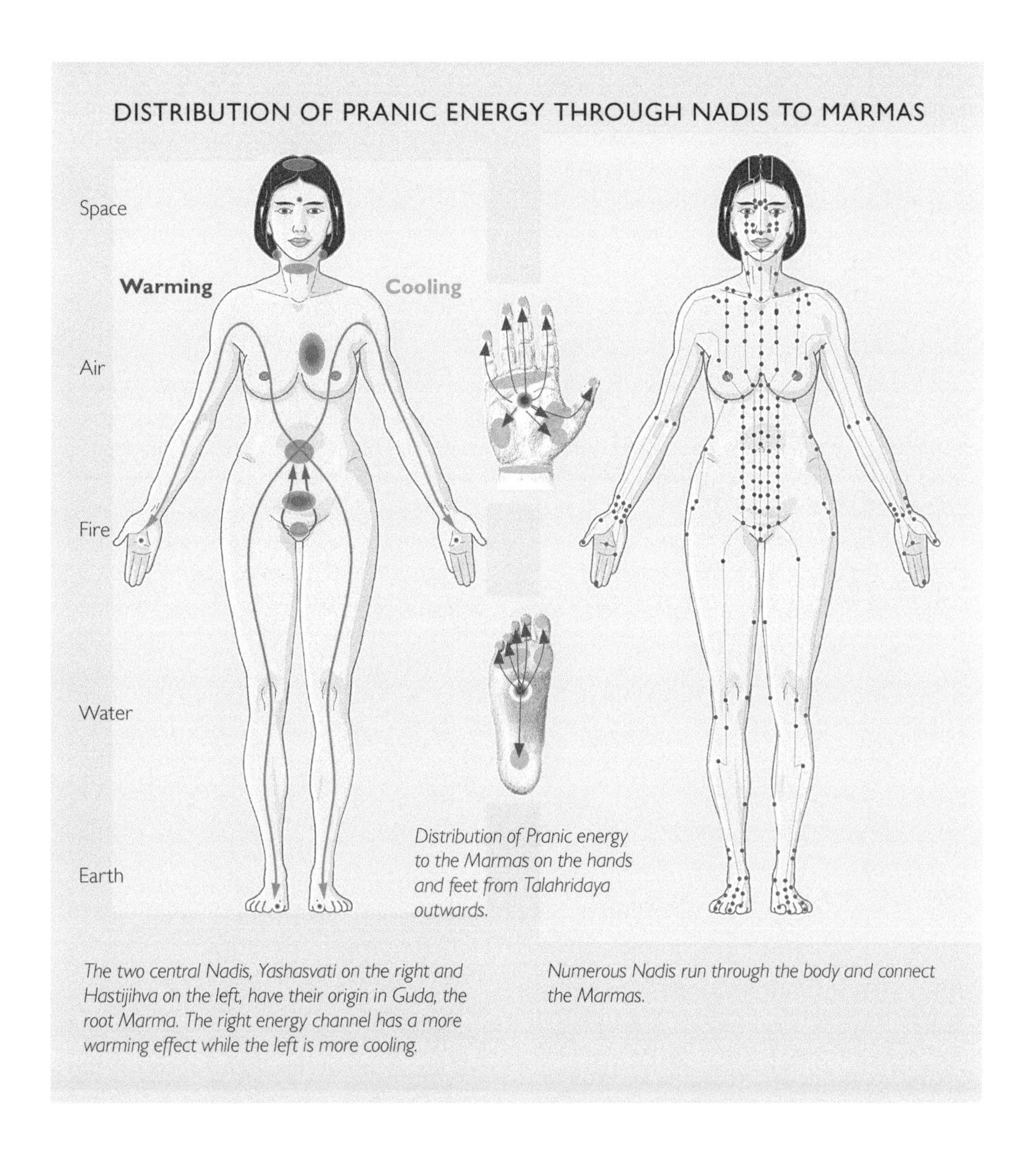


*Distribution of Pranic energy to the Marmas on the hands and feet from Talahridaya outwards.*

*The two central Nadis, Yashasvati on the right and Hastijihva on the left, have their origin in Guda, the root Marma. The right energy channel has a more warming effect while the left is more cooling.*

*Numerous Nadis run through the body and connect the Marmas.*

## The Marmas between the fingers – Kshipra

Kshipra means 'quick' because it has a fast effect in a treatment but also because it calms down movements that are too fast, such as convulsions. It is a tendon Marma and provides resilience and resistance.

**Application:** **Dissolving cramps (bronchial spasm in asthma, excitability with cramps), stimulation of lymphatic flow, colds, sore throat, pharyngitis, tonsillitis, laryngitis, sinusitis, neck tension, arm pain, shoulder pain, constipation, pain in general, Vata disorders, nervous exhaustion, depression from exhaustion, thyroid disorders.**

**Significance:** Kshipra sits in the 'webbing' between the fingers. It is an important and also easily accessible tendon Marma with a particular connection to the lymphatic system, the respiratory organs, maxillary sinuses, throat, tonsils, cervical spine, shoulder, colon and nervous system. Kshipra is responsible for rapid movement and quick thinking, and it activates memory. We snap our fingers if we have to remember something quickly.

**Control function:** The Kshipra between the thumb and index finger is the Sangam, the confluence of the energy pathways of the large intestine and lungs. Its centre is the point Large Intestine 4 of TCM. It is a so-called source point, has a strong connection with Prana (respiratory and nervous systems), strengthens the immune system, calms Vata, soothes pain, opens the large intestine meridian, acts on the face (eyes, nose, mouth and ears) and is traditionally used for colds, sweating, fever, facial paralysis, face- and headaches, dental pain, swelling and eye diseases. Secondary Kshipra areas are located in the webbing of the other fingers where the reflexology zones for the lymphatic organs are found. In the centre of the Kshipras are the so-called Baxie points of TCM.

**Immediate effect:** Relaxation of the back of the hand and the muscles in the neck on the same side, freer breathing through the nostrils, possible eructation, flowing sensations in the area of the inner or outer neck, relaxation in the lower abdomen.

**How to find Kshipra on the hand:** The main area of Kshipra is between the thumb and the index finger, extending from the outside to the inside of the hand. The secondary Kshipra points lie analogously between the other fingers.

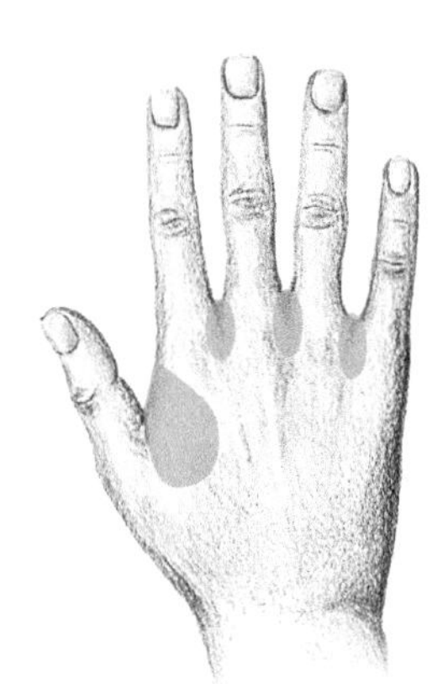

### OVERVIEW

**Marma type:** Snayu (tendon Marma)

**4 points:** 1 on each hand and 1 on each foot. Central Marma: Nila/Manya, communicates with Apalapa and Lohitaksha of the arm

**Effects:** controls lymph organs of the neck and especially the respiratory tract, sinus, tonsils and ear, and the upward movement of Vata (Udana); has influence on the large intestine, salivary glands (Bodhaka); nourishes the heart (Sadhaka) and strengthens the upper back (Avalambaka)

**Oils:** Vata massage oil for relaxation; for colds: MA 634 mint oil, Kapha massage oil, Kapha aroma oil, frankincense oil

**Adhimarma:** Udana, Adiprana

Self-treatment

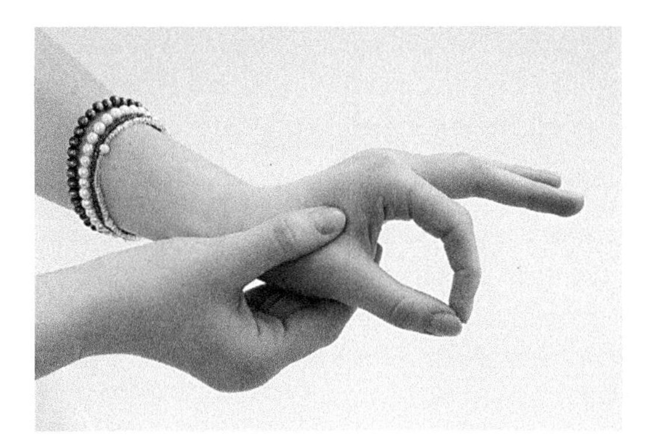

**Circular massage:** Sit comfortably and upright. Form the Gyan Mudra with the index finger and the thumb, as shown in the figure (see also page 114), and then massage with slight pressure using the thumb. The index, middle and ring fingers are placed on the counterpoint on the inside of the hand and they can gently participate in the massage movement.

To finish, gently massage the other Kshipra points in the 'webbing' between the fingers with your thumb and index finger using slightly stronger up-and-down movements.

Unless otherwise indicated, the 1–3–5–7 treatment format (see page 34) applies here, as with all other Marmas.

**Treatment time:** 2–3 minutes each hand.

Partner treatment

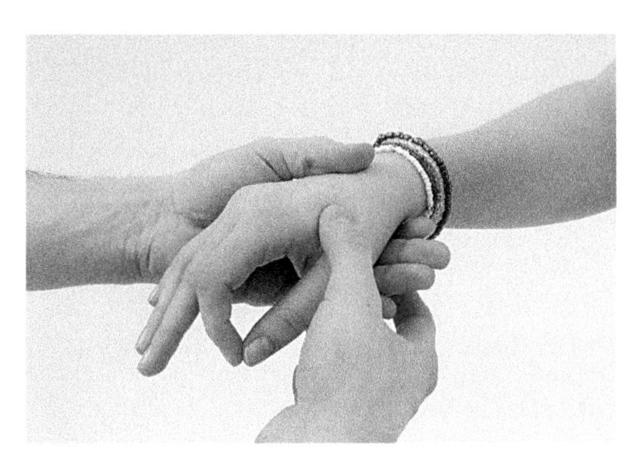

This is performed in the same way as the self-treatment. Your partner should also form the Gyan Mudra.

**Contact:** Hold your partner's hand from underneath with your left hand and place the palm of your right hand over the Marma to soothe and support it.

## The heart of the hand – Talahridaya

Talahridaya literally means 'the heart of the hand'. It is the centre of the palm, a muscle Marma. It stores energy and distributes it.

**Application: Nervousness and restlessness, exhaustion, grief, sorrow, indigestion, pain or stiffness in the hand, nervous heart complaints, circulatory disturbances.**

**Significance:** Talahridaya is the ordering and feeling intelligence of the hand, the peripheral Marma of the heart itself, and it presides over the energy of transformation (called Agni in Ayurveda). Through Talahridaya we share our emotions and life energy with our environment. When we reach out our hand to someone in greeting, our heart Marmas touch each other and interact. In classical Indian dance, one of the expressions of Gandharva Veda (Vedic music therapy), Talahridaya has an important role as the Marma of the heart and of love and is marked (see illustration on page 110).

**Control function:** The central hand Marma is the outpost of the heart Marma, which is the seat of the government of all the Marmas. From here, Prana is distributed into the five fingers. What we touch in the outside world is noticed by Talahridaya and this information is then forwarded to the heart Marma and all the other larger and smaller Marmas. All the hand meridians are in contact with Talahridaya, so it affects all bodily functions in the upper part of the body and in the digestive system.

**Immediate effect:** Soothing effect, perception of warmth in the belly, greater clarity of mind and stimulates flow of Prana, which is experienced as mental enlivenment and a feeling of freshness and opening in nasal breathing.

**How to find Talahridaya on the hand:** The Marma is exactly in the middle of the palm. Its support point is at the back of the hand, just opposite. The picture shows the hands of the dancer (illustration page 110) where the fingertips are also marked in red; these are also Marmas that are associated with feeling.

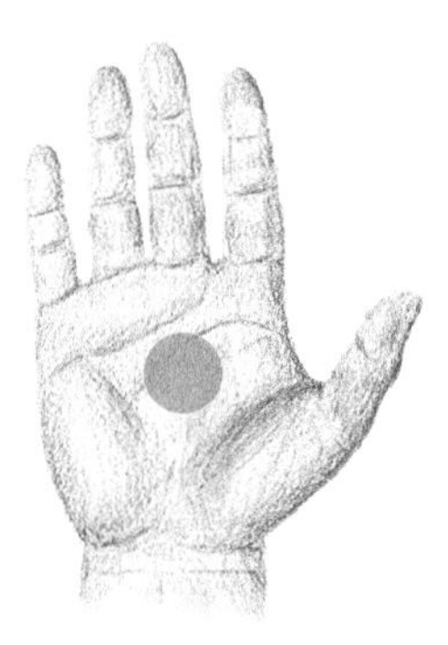

### OVERVIEW

**Marma type:** Mamsa (muscle Marma)

**4 points:** 1 point each on the left and right palm and on the sole of each foot

**Central Marma:** Hridaya

**Effects:** governs the emotions, stores energy and conserves strength; controls the heart's ability to feel and sense both inner and outer reality (Sadhaka), digestive power (Agni, Pachaka), circulation (Vyana) and Prana

**Oils:** Vata massage oil for calming, cinnamon, rose, jasmine, lotus, Vata aroma oil

**Adhimarma:** Hridaya

Self-treatment

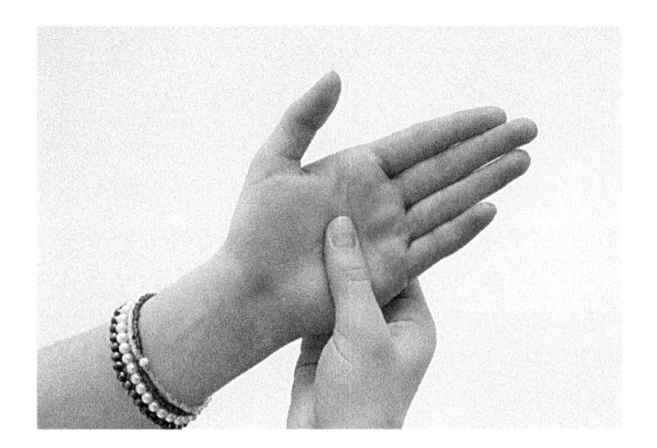

**Circular massage:** Sit comfortably and upright. Hold the hand to be treated so that the thumb lies on the Marma and the other fingers support the counterpoint on the back of the hand. Massage only with gentle pressure in a clockwise direction.

**Treatment time:** 3–5 minutes each hand.

Partner treatment

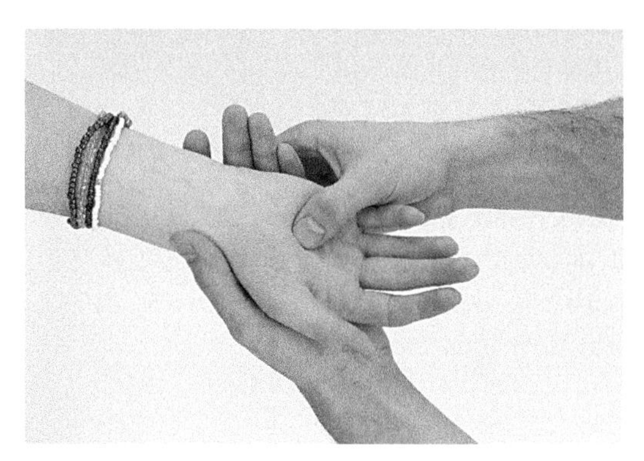

This is performed in the same way as self-treatment. Hold your partner's hand, palm upwards, with your left hand underneath their hand – this provides comfort and security. Then with your right thumb gently massage the Marma.

**Contact:** Hold your partner's upwards-facing palm with your left hand underneath and the right hand above, giving love, silence and security.

## The wrist Marma – Manibandha

Manibandha means 'that which connects the hand' (with the arm). As a joint Marma it monitors movement and stands for flexibility.

**Application:** **Vata disorders, tension in the wrist, general joint pain and a tendency to arthritis, neck and back pain, mental fatigue, weakness of concentration, insomnia, nervousness, bronchial asthma, tinnitus, carpal tunnel syndrome, stress-induced bowel dysfunction.**

**Significance:** Manibandha covers the whole wrist. It includes three smaller points inside and three more on the outside of the wrist. The central point (Bindu) is on the inside of the wrist, at the junction of the radius and carpal bones. In the wrist are located sensitivity, quick thinking, creativity and cheerfulness. There is a German saying, 'etwas locker aus dem Handgelenk schütteln', which means, literally, 'it is easy for someone to shake it out of the wrist', meaning that someone can create and express new ideas spontaneously and fluently. This conveys the specific qualities of the consciousness of the wrist Marma.

**Control function:** At least six energy channels pass through the wrist, three on the outside and three on the inside, for Vata, Pitta and Kapha; these are all coordinated by the wrist Marma. Amongst other areas, they connect with the lungs, heart, circulation, colon, small intestine, the endocrine system, eyes, teeth, ears, shoulders, neck and back. Thus the respiratory system (Prana, Udana), endocrine system (Shukra), cardiovascular functions (Vyana, Sadhaka) and the general suppleness of joints (Shleshaka) are all controlled by Manibandha.

Three other important Marma points are located here: the pulse-reading spots for Vata, Pitta and Kapha in the pulse of the radial artery.

**Immediate effect:** Calming of the mind, inner recollection, general relaxation, relaxation in the wrist, neck and back.

**How to find Manibandha:** Hold the wrist so that the thumb lies across the lines of the wrist. The thumb now covers the inside Marma completely. The index finger is on the corresponding outer support points of the wrist Marmas. Together they form the wrist Marma.

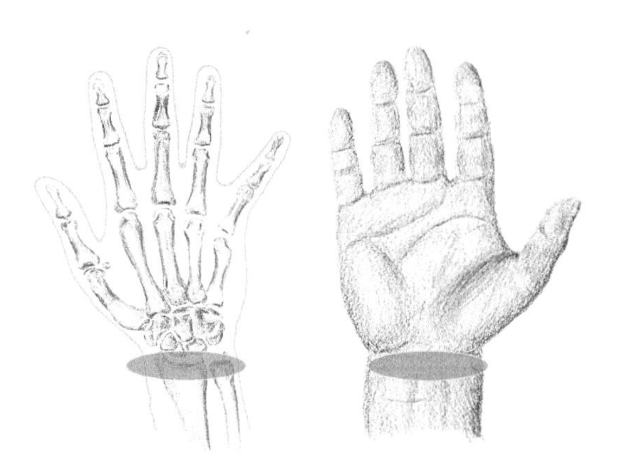

### OVERVIEW

**Marma type:** Sandhi (joint Marma)

**2 points:** 1 point on each arm

**Central Marma:** Hridaya

**Effects:** controls all three Doshas, but especially Vata; controls lubrication of the joints (Shleshaka), circulation (Vyana), feelings (Sadhaka), respiratory organs (Prana, Udana) and digestion (Pachaka); strengthens bones (Asthi), back and spine (Avalambaka); soothing effect for the ears (tinnitus)

**Oils:** ghee, Pitta oil, rose (with sensations of heat in the joint, Pitta disorders); Vata massage oil, lavender (calming); rosemary (stimulates circulation).

**Adhimarma:** Shanti Om, Sushumna, Mahaojas, Hridaya, Nidra

Self-treatment

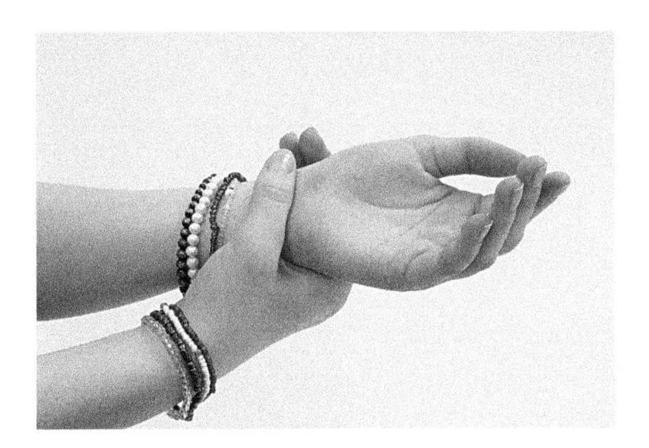

**Base position and circular massage:** Sit in a comfortable upright position. Breathe calmly and deeply in and out once through your nose. Hold the wrist so that the thumb lies across the lines of the wrist (as shown above). This is the base position.

The thumb pad is now on the central point (Bindu). The index, middle, ring and little fingers lie opposite, on the outside. Now, instead of massaging with the thumb, simply rotate the wrist between thumb and fingers back and forth. In this way you can massage all the points of Manibandha Marma around the wrist conveniently.

You can use the 1–3–5–7 format, or feel free to treat according to how you feel.

**Base position and Manibandha Mudra:** After each cycle, come back to the base position and rest on the Marma for one or two breaths. Relax the hand that you are holding and let it fall back loosely. Feel the calmness and relaxation that appear in the mind and body.

This base position acts like a Mudra. It develops the ability of letting go mentally and gives peace and confidence. You can also use it for yourself for relaxation and inner peace, as often as you like. In the evening it will help you to settle down and go to sleep.

**Treatment time:** 1–3 minutes each wrist.

Partner treatment

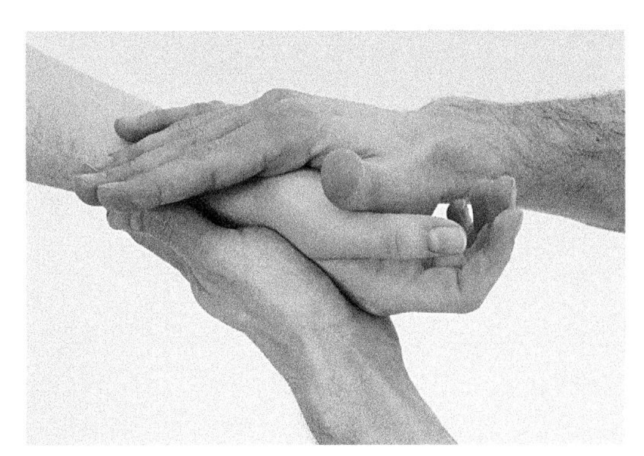

**Contact:** Hold the wrist with both hands as if you want to protect it and give comfort. Stay for a moment in this resting position (see above).

**Circular massage around the wrist:** Now let your palms slide smoothly in circular movements around your partner's wrist. Repeat the process several times and then switch to the other hand. This feels particularly enjoyable and relaxing for sensitive Vata types.

## The forearm Marma – Indrabasti

The Indrabasti Marma on the arm is the equivalent of the Marma on the calf with the same name (pages 62–63). It is a muscle Marma; it stores energy and transmits power. According to Indian mythology, Indra, the Lord of the Gods, lives on Mount Meru. He rides on a white elephant and is dressed in red.

**Application: Indigestion, constipation, stomach and intestinal cramping, circulatory weakness, mental fatigue, sexual weakness, bladder weakness, arm pain.**

**Significance:** Indrabasti monitors freedom of choice and helps us to keep our life under control, to be masters of our destiny. As a muscle Marma it stores energy and gives strength to the upper body area. It also acts on the bladder and sexual organs. Often this point can be slightly painful and tense if the flow of energy along the circulation meridian (Pericardium in TCM) going through it is blocked.

**Control function:** Indrabasti is one of the intermediary stations on the arm between the Mahamarmas and their representatives on the hand. At this point, nourishing Ojas connects with Vata, which brings energy upward (Udana); this process is supported by the nervous system (Tarpaka). This Marma communicates and mediates between the hand and the upper body Marmas via different energy pathways connecting the hands with the head and upper body.

**Immediate effect:** Relaxation in the arm and the neck; heat generation (Agni) in general but especially in the area of the bladder and sexual organs.

**How to find Indrabasti on the arm:**
The area of this Marma is located in the upper third of the inner forearm, right where the two forearm muscles make the shape of a peak, while creating a gap. The supporting counterpoint is directly opposite this area on the outer side of the forearm.

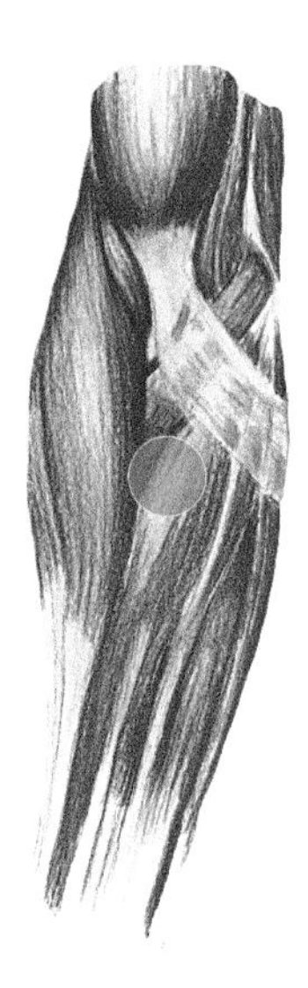

### OVERVIEW

**Marma type:** Mamsa (muscle Marma)

**4 points:** 1 point on each forearm and on each calf

**Central Marma:** Basti

**Effects:** gives strength, stores energy, controls digestive fire (Agni) and the power of digestion in the stomach and small intestine (Pachaka); connects Ojas with Udana-Vata, supported by Tarpaka-Kapha; strengthens mind power Prana and opens the flow of Vyana (distributing energy of the body)

**Oil:** Vata massage oil for relaxation; for arm pain MA 628 joint oil; for hormone disorders saffron and sandalwood

**Adhimarma:** Indrabasti

Self-treatment

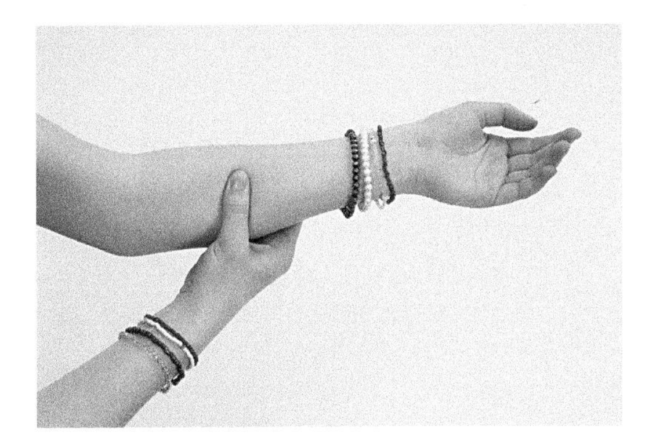

**Circular massage:** Sit comfortably and upright. Locate the point with the thumb on the inside of the forearm, approximately in the upper third. It is slightly sensitive to pressure. Place the thumb on the point, as shown in the illustration, and hold the forearm so that the index, middle and ring fingers come together on the counterpoint on the outside of the forearm. This area may also be slightly sensitive to pressure, especially if there is tension and pain in the neck and upper back.

Now massage gently and carefully in a circular motion using the thumb and the three fingers on the other side. If you press harder, it will take on the character of acupressure, which is more suitable for Kapha persons. For Vata people this Marma should only be treated with the flat hand, circling gently and sensitively in order to calm and harmonize.

This massage can also be performed on the opposite point on the outside of the forearm. This is particularly effective for tennis elbow.

**Treatment time:** 3–5 minutes each side.

Partner treatment

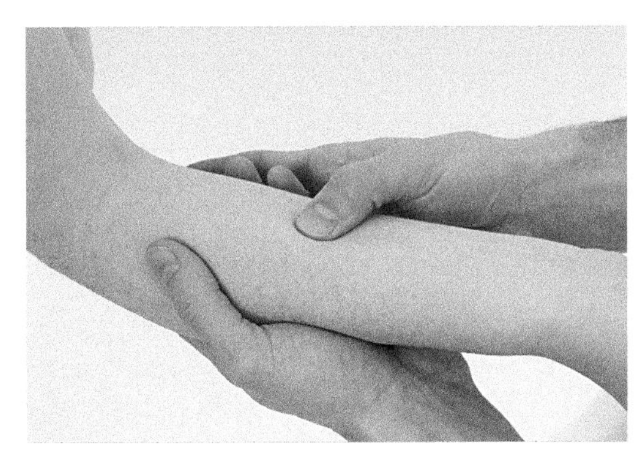

**Contact:** Hold the forearm on the opposite of Indrabasti with your left hand, gently place the right hand flat on the Marma and let peace, energy and heat flow for a few moments into the Marma.

**Circular massage:** Hold the forearm, as shown in the figure, with your left hand, and let your partner's arm rest in your hand. Massage gently and evenly clockwise with your thumb. Your other hand protects and strengthens the counterpoint and increases the effect on the Marma. Treat the point with feeling and attention. A sense of well-being should be generated; pain must never be caused. In very sensitive Vata people, massage the Marma with the flat hand.

The counterpoint on the outside of the forearm is particularly effective in arm pain. Treat it in the same way, but with the flat hand.

## The elbow Marma – Kurpara

Kurpara means 'elbow'. It is a joint Marma.

**Application: Tennis elbow, gastrointestinal disorders, circulation problems, depression, chest pain, trembling of the hands, pain in the neck, shoulder and back, aggression, cough, bronchial asthma.**

**Significance:** Kurpara covers the whole joint. There are important points covered by this Marma at the outer portion of the joint and inside the elbow. It is not just complaints caused by a physical overload that manifest themselves in the elbow (such as, for example, the typical 'tennis elbow'); inner conflict can also lead to tension and pain in this joint: there may, on the one hand, be an existential desire to liberate oneself from an uncomfortable situation and we make space for ourselves with the elbow, while on the other hand one may be expected to control oneself and behave considerately.

In addition to Vata, which means the movement in the joint, the elbow also has Pitta qualities as a 'sharp weapon'.

**Control function:** Like the wrist joint, Kurpara Marma encloses the circulation, lung and small intestine energy channels on the inner part of the elbow. In the outer part run the triple heater, colon and small intestine meridians. This explains its wide-ranging effects on the respiratory tract, stomach, intestine and cardiovascular system, on shoulder and arm pain as well as pain in the back of the neck, on overstimulation of the nervous system, or lack of *joie de vivre*.

**Immediate effect:** The treatment generally calms and reduces tension in the forearm muscles and also in the shoulder area and shoulder blades.

**How to find Kurpara:** Kurpara is the entire area around the elbow, front and back. If you hold the joint from the inside with the whole hand, then the tips of your middle and ring fingers are placed directly on one of the main points of Kurpara. This is also the painful area in tennis elbow.

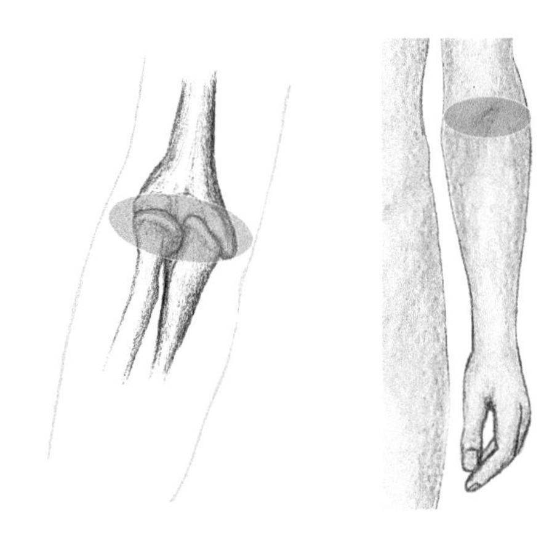

### OVERVIEW

**Marma type:** Sandhi (joint Marma)

**2 points:** 1 point on the left and 1 on the right arm

**Central Marma:** Hridaya

**Effects:** soothes nervous heart complaints (Sadhaka), calms the nerves (Prana), harmonizes the circulation (Vyana), relaxes the pelvis (Apana), strengthens digestion (Pachaka, Ranjaka), makes joints smooth (Asthi) and lubricates them (Shleshaka)

**Oil:** Vata massage oil, joint soothe oil, MA 628 joint oil

**Adhimarma:** Sushumna, Mahaojas, Shanti Om

## Self-treatment

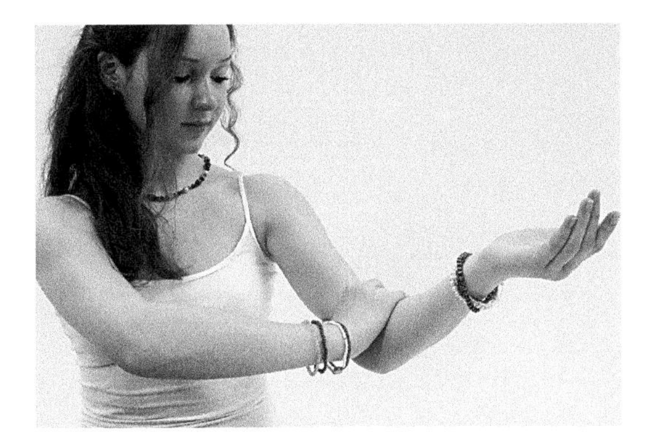

**Circular massage:** Hold the elbow with the hand from the inside and front of the elbow and slowly and gently massage the front of the joint in a circular movement; then let your hand rest still on the Marma (see illustration).

**Cross massage:** Now perform about 10 to 20 faster transverse massage movements from the front to the back of the elbow joint.

**Downward massage:** If you are suffering from 'tennis elbow' then also use the following massage treatment. Do three circles on the joint and then slide the hand down the arm towards the wrist, smoothing away the stress. Repeat this process until you feel clear relief.

**Treatment time:** 3–5 minutes each elbow.

## Partner treatment

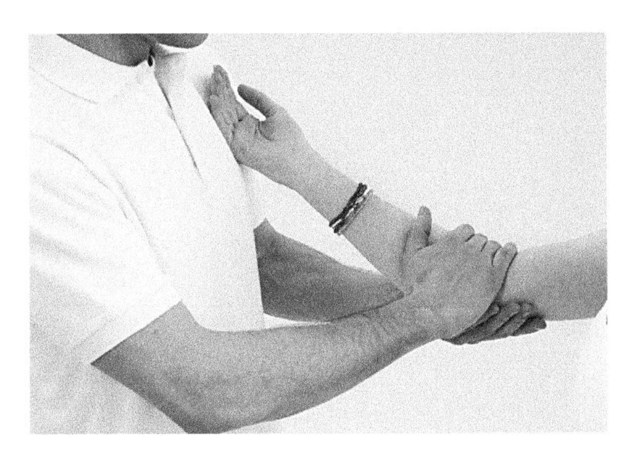

Partner treatment is done in the same way as self-treatment. Support the elbow joint with one hand from below. In the cross massage, lead with the fingers; in the circling movement, massage softly and calmly with the palm of the hand in oval movements on the front of the elbow.

Physiotherapists and masseurs sometimes use firm cross massages in tennis elbow (friction massages). The gentle, circular and then downward massage with joint soothe oil, however, often has quicker results in dissolving muscle tension, opening the energy flow in the meridians, and calming or eliminating irritation in the muscle attachment.

After oil application, always apply a hot, moist towel, which is very pleasing and soothing for the patient. Several sessions, preferably on consecutive days, may be required.

**Contact:** Hold the elbow as shown in the figure above and let your hands rest for a short time on the Marma before you start the massage treatment.

## Further Marmas on the arm

In the hand, upper arm, armpit and shoulder we find further important Marmas.

### The heel of the hand Marmas – Kurcha and Kurchashira

Kurcha means 'nodes' or 'bundles' (of muscles and tendons), and it refers to the hand muscles and tendons, especially on the thumb. The second Marma, Kurchashira, means the head (*Shira*) of the muscle and sinew bundle on the thumb. The two tendon Marmas relate to weak vision, eye disease, hormonal disorders and thyroid disorders. The influence of Kurcha and Kurchashira on vision is somewhat difficult to understand at first. But if we look at the reflex zones on the hand we find the larger part of the two Marmas on the so-called mount of Venus. It is the whole area of the thenar eminence. This will help us explain the connection between this area, eyesight and hormones. During the menopause the production of female sex hormones declines, particularly oestrogen. During this transition phase the muscle often shrinks, arthrosis in the joint of the thumb can develop and the eyesight deteriorates, usually in the direction of long-sightedness. The Subdosha for vision is Alochaka. It also represents hormone regulation by the pituitary gland. Furthermore, in hyperthyroidism the eye may be affected, for example in Graves' disease.

Treat the two heels of the hand Marmas in the same way as Talahridaya (pages 46–47). If there is pain in the thumb base joint and the heel of the hand, massage it with MA 628 joint oil.

### The upper arm Marma – Ani

Ani means the 'point of a nail'. In Vedic times it was also the axle of a wheel in vehicles. There is a front point (figure 1 (a)) lying on the transition of the biceps muscle to its tendon, and a rear one (b) on the aponeurosis of the triceps muscle. The main applications of this tendon Marma are arm pain, fluid retention (oedema), poor circulation, and kidney and pancreatic disease. The point on the biceps muscle can be treated with the flat hand or from underneath, by embracing it with the thumb (photos 2, 3). In partner treatment, one hand supports from beneath the triceps point; the other gently massages from the top. You can also use both thumbs to massage (photos 4, 5). Use soothing, analgesic, relaxing oils for muscle tension and arm pain, for example joint soothe oil, or for oedema use diuretic oils such as juniper.

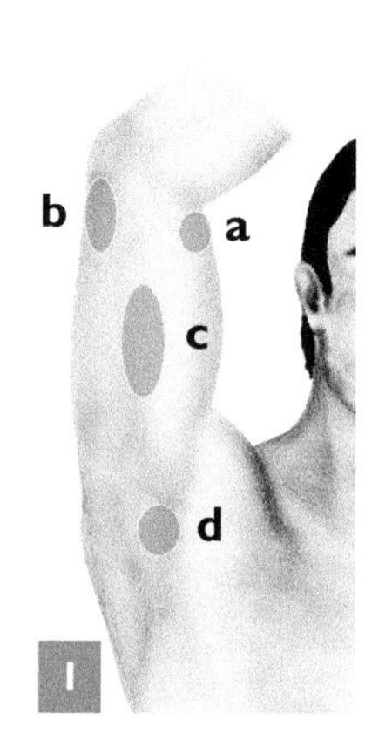


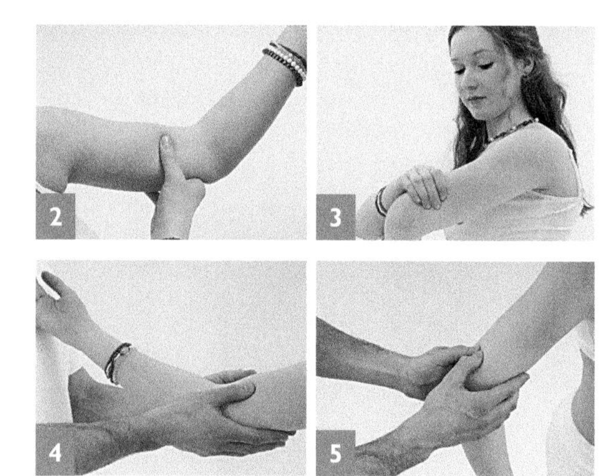

## The vascular Marma on the upper arm – Urvi or Bahvi

Like Ani Marma, *Urvi* (figure 1 (c), page 54) controls water balance as well as the circulatory system. As a vascular Marma it also moves heat, Agni, to the thoracic organs. Urvi is easy to find. Grip the middle of the upper arm from above so that the thumb is on the inside (photo 1). If you touch a little deeper, through the muscle, then you can feel the brachial artery pulsating. The main point of the Marmas is right here. Do the treatment several times, very gently, ideally with a flat hand (photo 2), using the 1–3–5–7 treatment format. Please do not use pressure, as this is not indicated for massaging blood vessels or muscles. We want to gently feel and enliven the field of consciousness of Urvi.

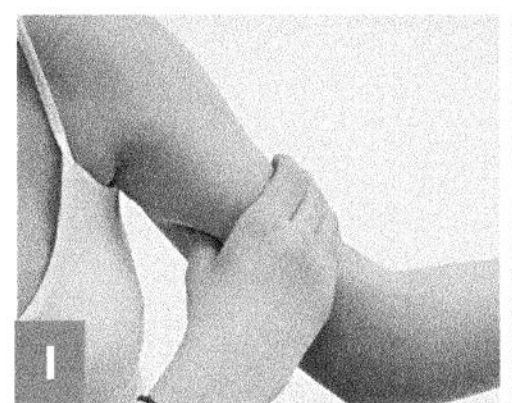

1

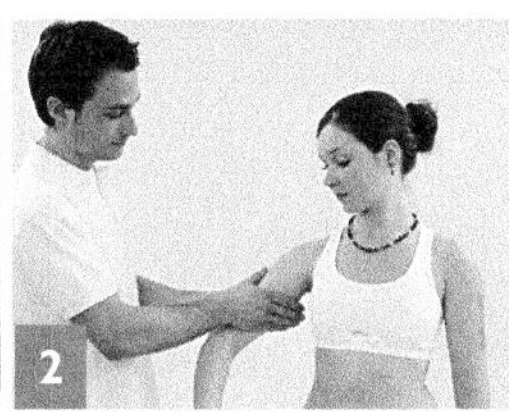

2

## The Marma of the armpit – Lohitaksha (arm)

This vascular Marma is exactly in the centre of the armpit, in the depth of which blood vessels, nerves and lymphatic ducts all merge (figure 1 (d), page 54). This is a very sensitive point that should only be treated with experience. Like Lohitaksha on the leg, which is located in the groin, the Marma controls the lymphatic system.

## The shoulder muscle Marma – Kakshadhara

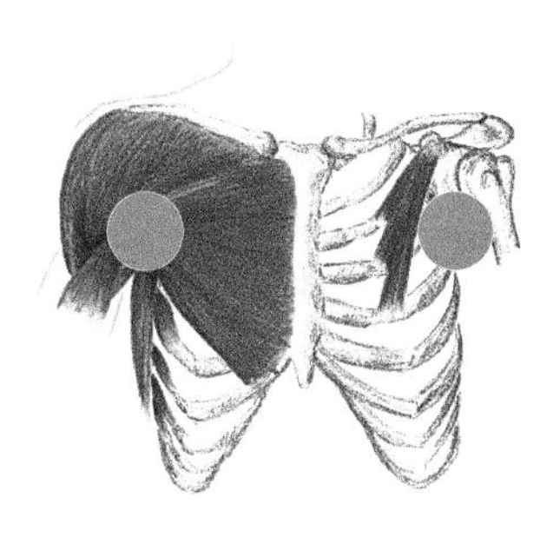

This tendon Marma is located in the pit created by the deltoid muscle and the chest, three finger-breadths under the clavicle. In the depth the coracoid process of the shoulder blade is palpable. This is the energetic connection point for the major and minor chest muscles, the lymphatic vessels, arteries and veins of the armpit, as well as the median nerve, which goes from the middle of the arm to the hand. At the coracoid process, thus completely around the centre of Kakshadhara, there is frequently pain at the attachment of the tendon, radiating to the shoulder, chest and lower neck. The three Doshas are present in this Marma in almost equal measure, with a slight emphasis on Kapha. Great relief can be gained from a gentle Marma massage using Vata calming oils, such as Vata massage oil, MA 628 joint oil, arnica, comfrey or clove. With the three fingers of the hand or thumb, we can easily reach the Marma and treat it beneficially (photos 3, 4). Also try the 1–3–5–7 treatment format here, or simply go by how you feel.

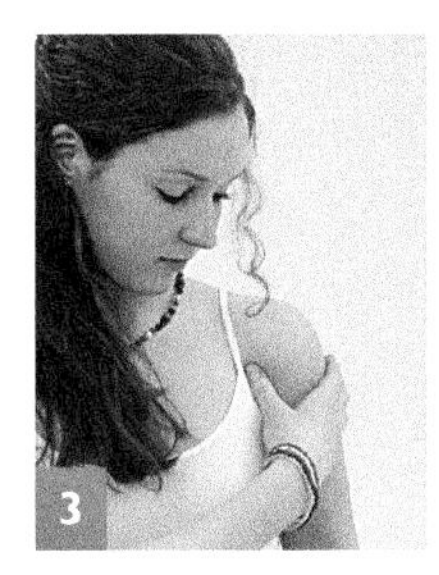

3

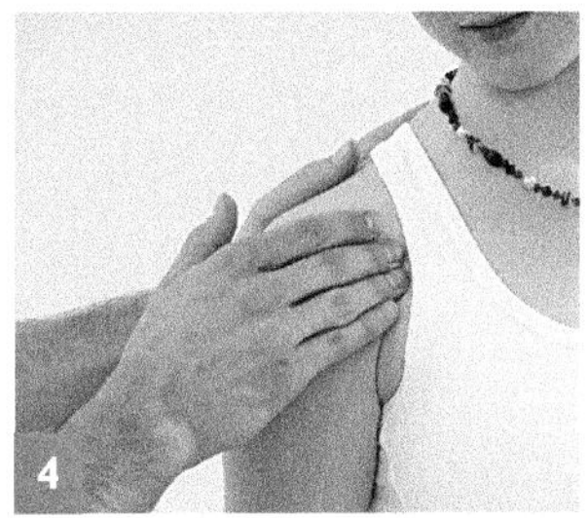

4

## The Marma between the toes – Kshipra

Kshipra means fast – in this case not only because it has an immediate effect in a treatment, but also because it calms down excessive excitation as well as fast movements such as convulsions. It is a tendon Marma that provides explosive strength and resilience (see also Kshipra Marmas between fingers Marma, pages 44–45).

**Application: Relieving cramp (foot and leg cramp, bronchospasm in asthma), stimulation of lymphatic flow, pain in the big toe, liver and gall bladder disease, colds and respiratory disorders, headache and toothache, urinary retention, sleep disorders, back pain, nervous heart complaints.**

**Significance:** In Kshipra Marma we find the consciousness that is related to a fast and exhilarating walk, jumping up, or standing on tiptoe. If we go through life elated, relaxed, natural and on our own two feet, then we remain in the flow. By walking barefoot we activate Kshipra, strengthen the lymph organs and digestive glands, and we stay healthy. Kshipra affects the strength of the back and our overall posture. A 'dancing' walk is only possible if we walk upright and think straight and, at the same time, such a walk enlivens these qualities within us.

**Control function:** Kshipra is found in the 'webbing' between the toes. It is an important and also easily accessible tendon Marma with a particular connection to the lymphatic system, which has reflex points on the Kshipra Marmas. The energy pathways of the stomach, liver, spleen, pancreas and bladder all run through this Marma. Like Kshipra on the hands, it also acts on the respiratory organs, sinuses, tonsils and the nervous system. It keeps the spine flexible and the heart elated.

**Immediate effect:** Relaxation in the lower back, increased alertness and freshness, relaxation of the soles of the feet, warmth and energy in the perineum.

**How to find Kshipra on the foot:** The main Marma lies in the gap between the big and the second toe on both the top and the underneath of the foot. Secondary Marmas are located analogously between the other toes.

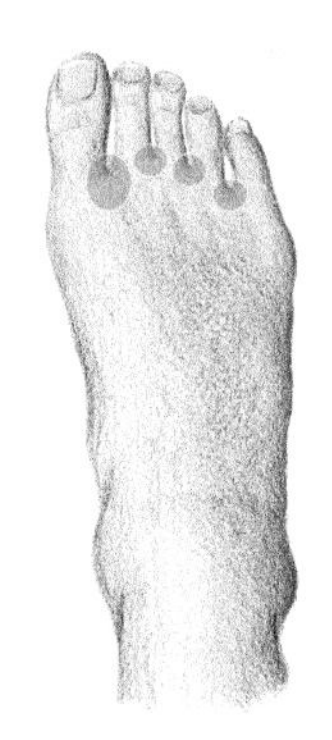

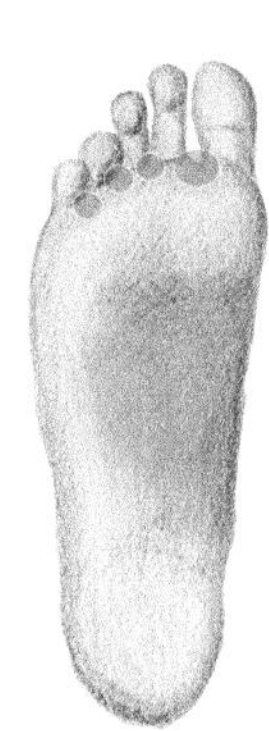

### OVERVIEW

**Marma type:** Snayu (tendon Marma)

**4 points:** 1 on each hand and 1 on each foot

**Central Marma:** Nila/Manya, communicates with Lohitaksha, Vitapa and Guda

**Effects:** controls the spleen, lymph organs in the pelvis and pancreas, liver, stomach, bladder, sinus, ear and tonsils, and the downward movement of Vata (Apana); it nourishes the heart (Sadhaka) and the lungs and strengthens the back (Avalambaka)

**Oils:** MA 628 joint oil, MA 634 mint oil (for respiratory problems); joint soothe oil, sesame (arthritis, pain in general); Vata oil, Vata aroma oil, lavender, valerian (anxiety, restlessness)

**Adhimarma:** Udana, Adiprana, Sushumna, Shanti Om

## Self-treatment

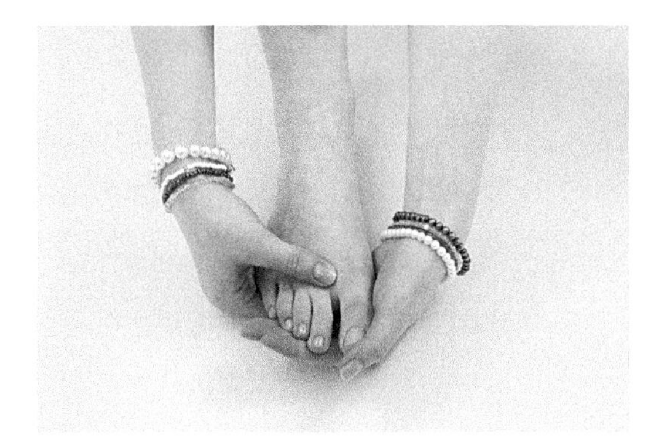

**Circular massage with the thumb:** Sit comfortably with bent knees. Embrace the foot with one hand from below and, using the thumb of the other hand, do oval massage movements between the first and second toe.

You can use the 1–3–5–7 treatment format or treat according to your own feeling and comfort.

**Up-and-down massage:** Massage the Marmas between all the toes with both thumbs, with one thumb moving up as the other moves down.

**Treatment time:** 2–3 minutes each foot.

## Partner treatment

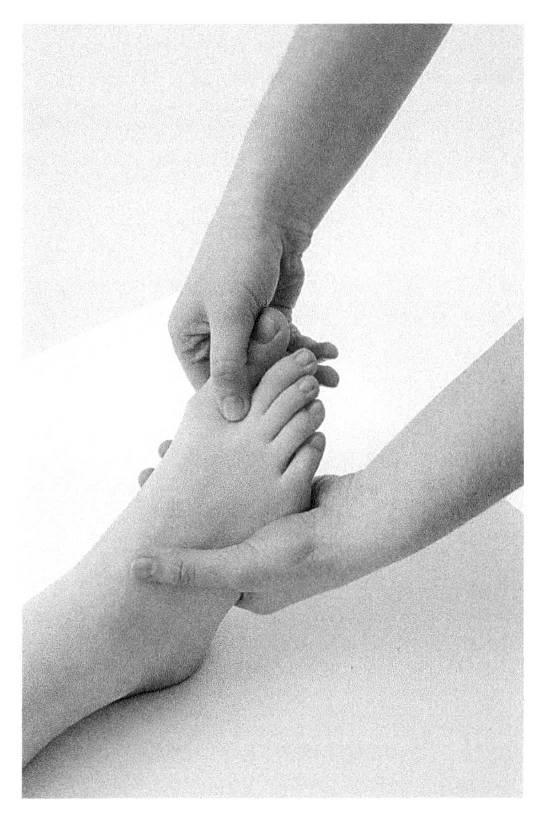

Your partner lies comfortably on their back. The treatment is analogous to self-treatment.

**Contact:** Embrace your partner's foot with your left hand underneath the foot and the right hand lying soothingly on top of the foot.

## The heart of the foot – Talahridaya

Talahridaya is situated in the centre of the sole of the foot, which is analogous to the position of Talahridaya of the hand (pages 46–47). As a muscle Marma it stores energy and distributes it.

**Application: Nervousness and restlessness, sleeping disorders, exhaustion, grief, sorrow, digestive weakness, pain or tension in the foot, nervous heart complaints, circulation disorders, kidney disease.**

**Significance:** Talahridaya is the ordering and sentient intelligence of the hand or foot, the peripheral Marma of the heart itself, and it controls the energy of transformation, which in Ayurveda is called Agni.

**Control function:** The heart Marma of the foot is a branch of the great heart Marma in the centre of the body. We could say that it represents the central government to the outside. It receives its energy through the Nadis which come from the heart and other central Marmas, especially the navel, bladder and root Marmas. Talahridaya then distributes this Prana to the five toes that grab hold and feel. From here contact with the ground, the earth, is also established and energetic information is fed back to the body via leading returning Nadis. This is one reason why it is so healthy to walk barefoot. All energy channels to the foot and back to the body have links to Talahridaya. It affects all body functions, especially in the lower body and in the digestive system. From Talahridaya of the foot we also drain out excessive Vata or toxins from the body. In its centre is the first point of the kidney meridian.

**Immediate effect:** Sedation, perception of warmth in the stomach, relaxation in the legs and pelvis, increased clarity of mind and flow of Prana, which is experienced as mental enlivenment.

**How to find Talahridaya on the foot:** The Marma is located a little above the centre of the sole of the foot. Its support point is on the back of the foot, just opposite.

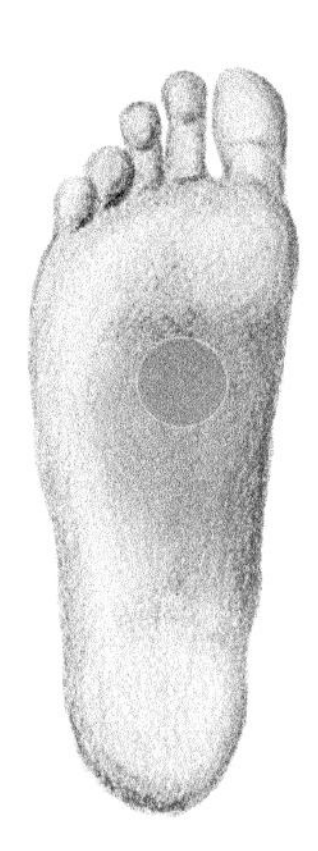

### OVERVIEW

**Marma type:** Mamsa (muscle Marma)

**4 points:** 1 point on each hand and 1 point on each foot

**Central Marma:** Hridaya

**Effects:** Hridaya controls digestive processes (Agni, Pachaka), stores energy and maintains strength; controls feeling and perception of heart (Sadhaka), circulation (Vyana) and Prana.

**Oils:** for calming – Vata massage oil, cinnamon, Ylang Ylang, Vata aroma oil; in hot flushes or heat in the legs: Pitta oil or ghee

**Adhimarma:** Hridaya, Nabhi

Self-treatment

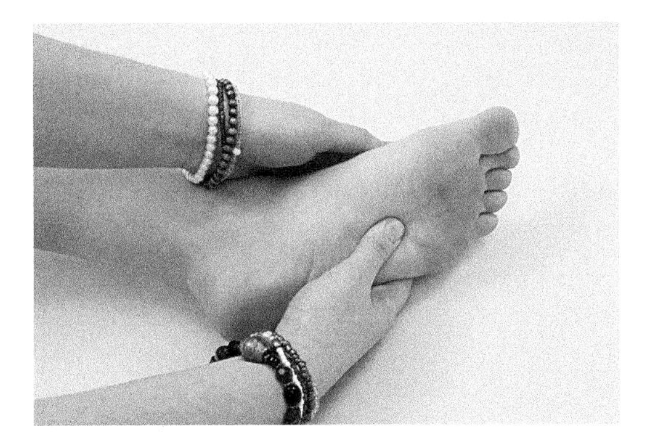

**Circular massage:** Sit comfortably. Embrace the foot to be treated with the hand so that the thumb is on the Marma and your other hand supports the opposite point on the back of the foot. Massage in a clockwise direction using only gentle pressure.

**Treatment time:** 3–5 minutes per foot.

Partner treatment

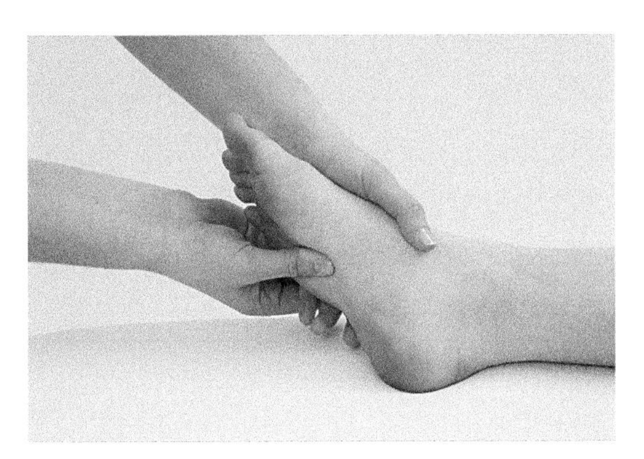

This is done in the same way as self-treatment. Your partner can lie comfortably on their back. You sit in front of their feet and massage the Marma from underneath with your thumb. With a little practice you can even massage the Marmas on both left and right foot at the same time. To do this, hold the feet with your fingers above the big toe and massage the Marmas with your thumbs circling in opposite directions. This feels extremely pleasant.

**Contact:** Embrace the foot with both hands, with palms on the Marma and its support point on the back of the foot, and give it warmth and rest for some moments.

## The ankle Marma – Gulpha

Gulpha means 'ankle'. It is a joint Marma.

**Application: Anxiety, mental and physical insecurity, lack of coordination in walking, disease of the pelvic organs, sexual disorders, tinnitus and eye strain, mental restlessness, sleeping disorders, restless leg syndrome.**

**Significance:** Gulpha monitors stability in life as well as in the foot itself. The Marma sits in the gap of the joint, and controls coordination and the sense of space in the ankle. It also regulates pressure distribution and the weight of the entire body on the feet. Anxiety, time pressure, hectic activity, insecurity, disregard for inner guidance, stubbornness and a Vata-aggravating diet (dehydration of the joints) can stress the Marma. Frequent twisting of one's ankle can happen not only in sport but also through lack of attention, when the spirit wants to move faster than the body is ready for.

**Control function:** Gulpha has a controlling influence over the kidney, spleen, pancreas and stomach meridians on the inside of the ankle and the bladder, liver and stomach meridians on the outside. In this way, the Marma coordinates powerful control points in the physiology, particularly sexuality, hormone regulation, digestive metabolism and fluid balance.

**Immediate effect:** Relaxation, increased mental peace and clarity, relaxation of the back, easing of the pelvis.

**How to find Gulpha:** The area of this Marma covers the ankle; its centre is on the inside, below and slightly forward of the lower end of the shin bone (tibia).

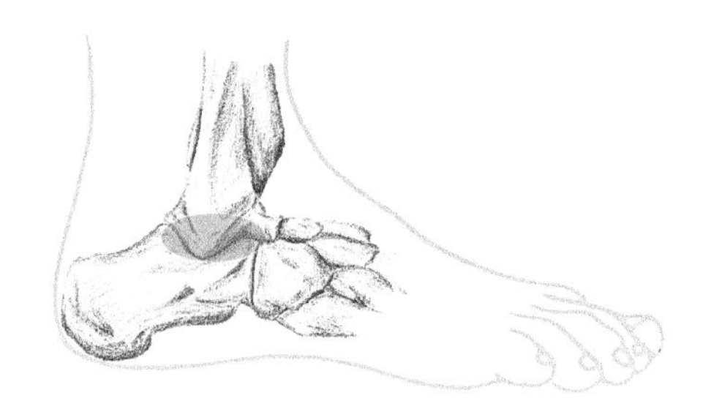

### OVERVIEW

**Marma type:** Sandhi (joint Marma)

**2 points:** 1 point on each ankle

**Central Marma:** Hridaya

**Effects:** controls joint fluids (Shleshaka); gives clear, calm thinking (Prana) and relaxes Apana (physical elimination, letting go mentally); controls sexual organs (Shukra), hormone regulation, digestive metabolism (Pachaka, Ranjaka) and fluid balance

**Oils:** MA 628 joint oil, joint soothe oil, sesame (arthritis, pain), Vata oil, lavender, valerian, Brahmi Taila (anxiety, restlessness), Ylang Ylang

**Adhimarma:** Gulpha, Basti, Nabhi, Sushumna, Shanti Om, Hridaya

## Self-treatment

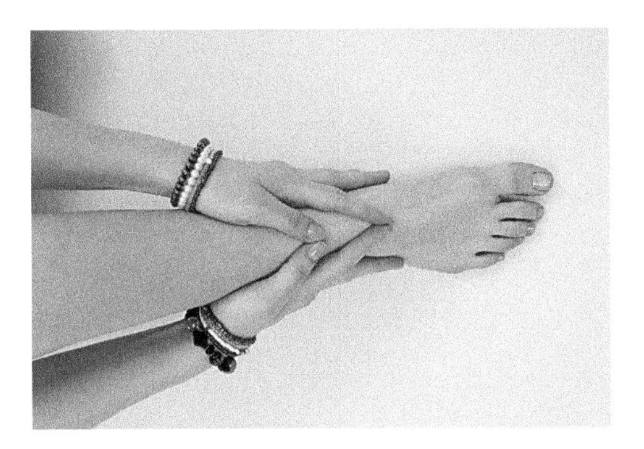

**Circular massage with both hands:** Sit comfortably with a slightly bent knee. Grasp the ankle with both hands, with your palms and fingers covering it gently. Now massage gently, using up-and-down movements, with the fingers moving around the inner and the outer ankle. In the downward movement the index finger and thumb are touching (see illustration); in the upward movement they open to the back. Repeat several times.

**Mudra for faith and stability:** Finish with the Mudra shown in the illustration and let the hands rest on the ankle for about one minute.

**Treatment time:** 2–3 minutes per ankle.

## Partner treatment

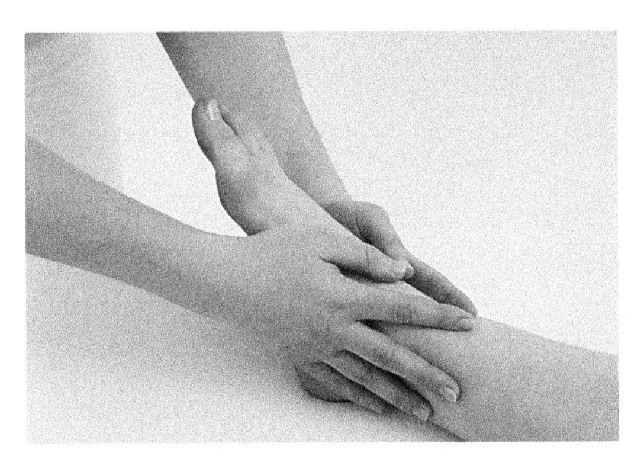

Your partner lies comfortably on their back, with the leg stretched out. The treatment is similar to self-treatment. Massage the ankle Marma especially gently. Again finish with the Mudra, as shown in the illustration.

**Contact:** For the left foot, the left hand is placed on the inner ankle, with the right on the outer ankle (and conversely for the right foot).

**Treatment time:** 2–3 minutes per ankle.

## The calf Marma – Indrabasti

**Application:** **Back pain, sciatica, tired legs, calf pain and tightness after over-exertion, calf cramps, sexual disorders, gynaecological problems, prostate problems, haemorrhoids, mental dullness, tired eyes, lymphedema in legs.**

**Significance:** Indrabasti watches over our freedom of decision. It allows us to have our life under control, to rule over our own life. This point is often painful and tense, with the energy flow along the bladder meridian blocked. As a muscle Marma it stores energy, gives strength and releases heat (see also 'The forearm Marma', pages 50–51).

**Control function:** The Marma communicates between the foot and the central Marmas of the body centre, especially Basti, the bladder Marma. Indrabasti is a confluence of energy pathways, principally of the bladder as well as the stomach and gall bladder. The centre of the Marma (Bindu) corresponds to the point Bladder 57 in TCM. For this reason, treatment of this point has a very special effect: stimulation of fluid secretion and relief of pain along the bladder meridian, including relief of back pain, sciatica and discomfort in the pelvic organs.

**Immediate effect:** Relief of tension in the lower back, sensation of a channel opening in the entire leg and even in the other leg or the arm (the Indrabasti of the arm), energy flow in the perineum and in the organs of the lower abdomen, general relaxation, opening sensation in the eyes.

**How to find Indrabasti on the leg:** The area of this Marma can be found precisely where the two calf muscles form a mountain peak. The Marma in its expanded form has the shape of a rhombus, and the bladder meridian, Basti Nadi, runs through its centre.

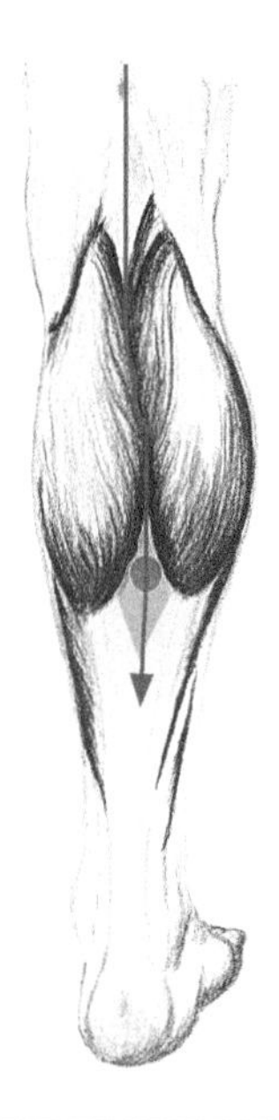

### OVERVIEW

**Marma type:** Mamsa (muscle Marma)

**4 points:** 1 on each leg and 1 on each arm

**Central Marma:** Basti

**Effects:** has Pitta and Vata properties; monitors excretion of urine (Apana), gives strength, stores energy, communicates with the feelings of the heart (Sadhaka), activates metabolism and digestive fire (Agni), digestive power (Pachaka) and transportation of food in the intestine (Samana); opens channels for distribution of pranic energy (Vyana); has connections to all areas of the body; opens the eyes

**Oils:** for relaxation – Vata oil, almond oil; for cooling in case of heat and other forms of Pitta – mint oil, Pitta oil, ghee

**Adhimarma:** Indra Royal

Self-treatment

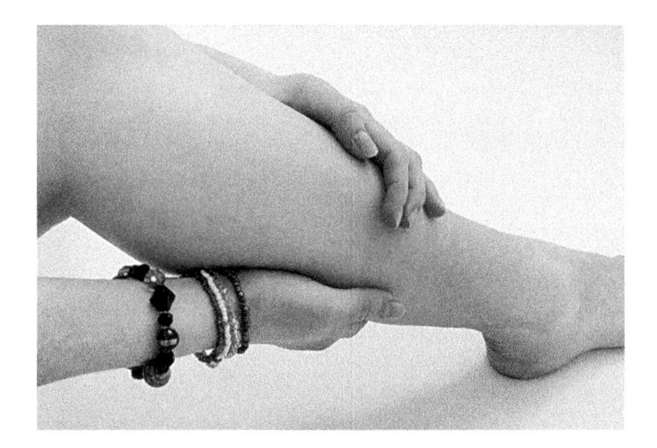

**Circular massage with the palm of the hand:** Sit comfortably and find the point indicated in the diagram using your fingertips. The Marma is slightly sensitive to pressure. Massage it gently. Vata people should massage this point very gently and sensitively with a circular motion and only with a flat hand. The other hand supports and protects the Marma on the opposite side on the shin. Massage the right calf clockwise and the left one anti-clockwise. Use the 1–3–5–7 treatment format and repeat 4 to 8 times.

**Gentle up-and-down strokes and stretching of the Marma:** Provided that the calf and the Marma are not oversensitive, then you can enclose the calf with both hands and massage with your fingertips from the bottom to the top along the middle of the calf, which is the energy path of the bladder meridian (see illustration on page 62), and back down on the sides. You open the Marma by gently pulling the point outwards on the calf using the fingertips, which allows the energy to flow. Stop after a few seconds and give the Marma about 10 seconds to rest. Repeat 4 to 8 times.

**Completion of treatment:** Finally massage once again in circles with the flat hand, bring the point to rest and let the treatment gently fade out.

**Treatment time:** 2–3 minutes per leg.

Partner treatment

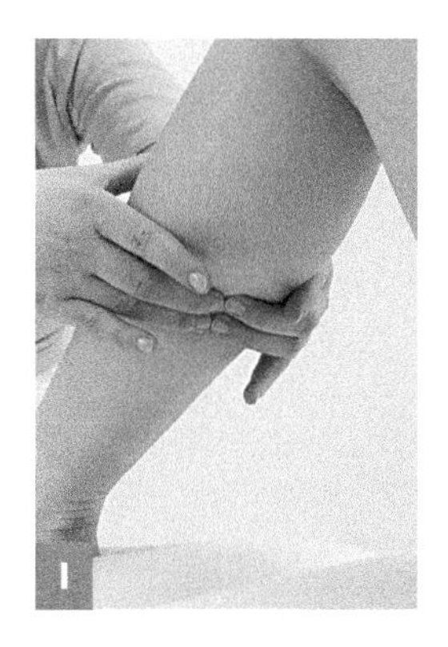
1

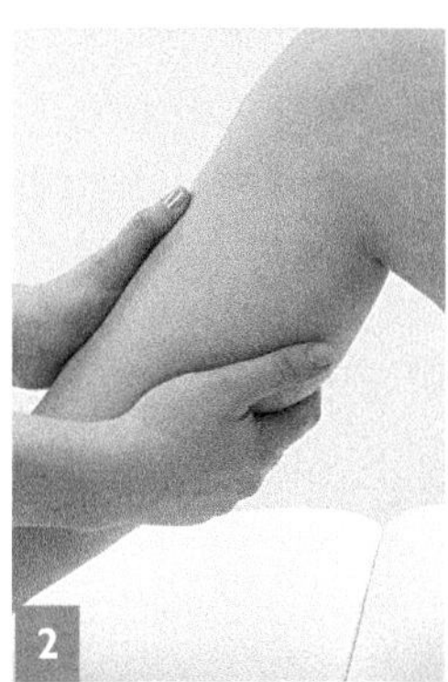
2

Ask your partner to lie comfortably on their back with bent knees. The treatment is similar to self-treatment. Treat the point with caution. A sense of well-being should be generated and there should not be any pain. Also be careful with varicose veins. Massage the area of the Marma with a flat hand or gently with the two middle fingers, holding the calf from the front (photo 1).

**Contact:** The right hand is on the calf; the left one is opposite on the shin (photo 2).

## The knee Marma – Janu

Janu means 'knee'; it is a joint Marma.

**Application: Knee pain, arthrosis/ arthritis, kneecap pain (chondropathia patellae), knee injury, anxiety, inner restlessness, nervousness, sleep disorders, liver and bile problems, biliary pain (right knee), spleen and pancreatic disorders (left knee).**

**Significance:** This joint Marma represents our awareness in the knee. When Pranic energy is strong here, we stand firmly in life; we are steadfast and settled within ourselves. If the Marma is weakened, especially if anxiety is the cause, our knees shake, we feel insecure and we lose physical stability. The same is true in a metaphorical mental sense.

**Control function:** The energy pathways of the bladder, kidney, liver, gall bladder, stomach, spleen and pancreas run through this Marma, so it has very important functions in the control of these organ systems. Its main task, however, is to ensure the stability of the joint and the mind.

**Immediate effect:** Peace and warmth in the knee joint, increase of general well-being, calmness and peace of mind.

**How to find Janu:** This Marma encompasses the entire knee, with its energy being particularly focused in the middle of the back of the knee and at the bottom of the kneecap. Smaller vital points sit around the kneecap and at the back of the knee.

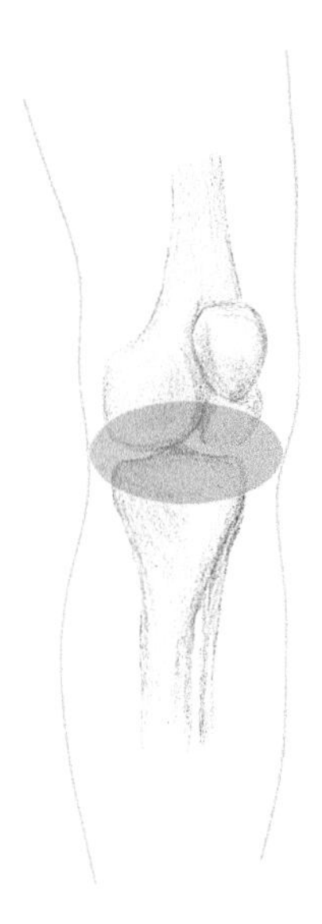

### OVERVIEW

**Marma type:** Sandhi (joint Marma)

**2 points:** 1 on each knee

**Central Marma:** Nabhi

**Effects:** coordinates the function and lubrication of joints (Shleshaka); controls energy flow to internal organs (liver, gall bladder, stomach, bladder, kidney, spleen, pancreas)

**Oils:** MA 3628 joint oil, joint soothe oil, sesame (arthritis, pain in general), Vata oil, Vata aroma oil, valerian, lavender, Brahmi Taila (anxiety, restlessness)

**Adhimarma:** Sushumna, Nabhi

### Self-treatment

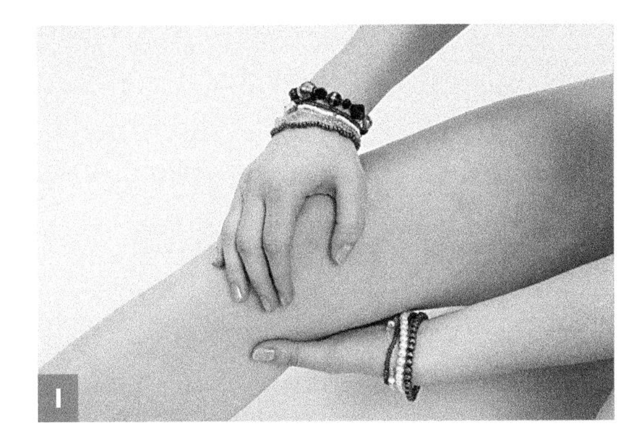

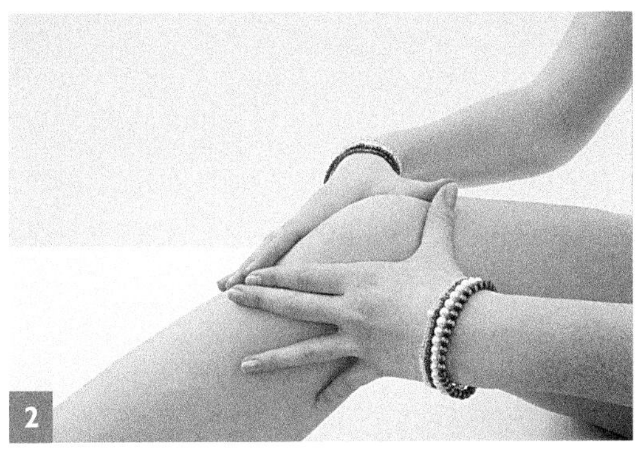

**Circular massage with the whole hand:** Sit comfortably with a slightly bent knee. Put the palm of your right hand on the kneecap, with the left on the back of the knee (photo 1). Massage gently in circles using the flat of the hand in a sensitive and calming manner. The other hand supports and protects the Marma at the back of the knee, and can also do circular massage movements, half a circle behind the upper hand. Massage the right knee in a clockwise direction and left knee anti-clockwise. This procedure also treats another leg Marma called Ani, which is about three to four fingers above the kneecap (page 66). Repeat the 1–3–5–7 treatment format 2 to 4 times.

**'The fox head' Mudra of the knee:** When finished, put your fingers and hands over the knee (photo 2). Make sure that the thumb, forefinger and middle finger touch each other, and the other fingers encompass the joint. Viewed from above, the Mudra has the form of a fox head. This has an excellent calming effect and brings Prana to the knee. Let the Mudra work for one to five minutes.

**Treatment time:** 3–5 minutes per knee.

### Partner treatment

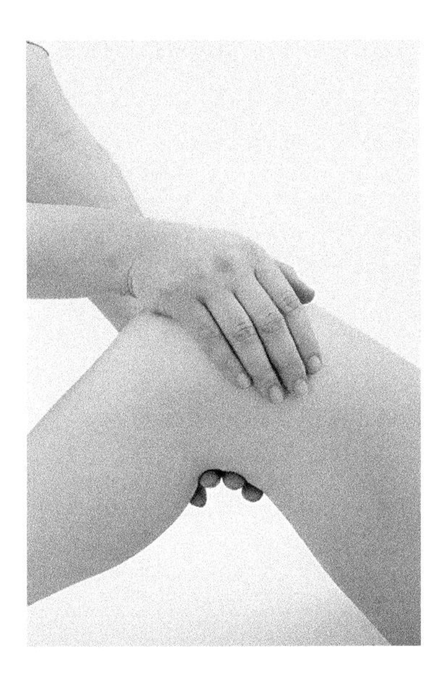

Ask your partner to lie comfortably on their back with the knee bent at 90 degrees. The treatment is similar to self-treatment. The treatment is very gentle and calm.

**Contact:** Left hand over the kneecap, with right hand at the back of the knee.

## Further Marmas on the leg

There are other important Marmas on the leg: on the foot, between the thigh and the groin and at the pubic bone.

### The ball of the foot Marma – Kurcha – and the heel Marma – Kurchashira

Kurcha extends from the muscle ball of the big toe across the muscles and tendons of the other toes (see diagram below). Kurchashira can be found at the attachment of the foot muscles to the heel, where we transfer power when we walk and run. It controls tension in the muscles in general, but especially in the leg. This Marma point is often slightly painful. The main application areas are visual impairment, endocrine disturbances and thyroid diseases; additional applications for Kurchashira are digestive weakness, sexual weakness, tired legs and feet, prostate problems, menstrual problems, mental tension, general muscle tension and back pain. Treat the two Marmas like Talahridaya (pages 58–59). Pitta cooling oils and ghee are mostly indicated.

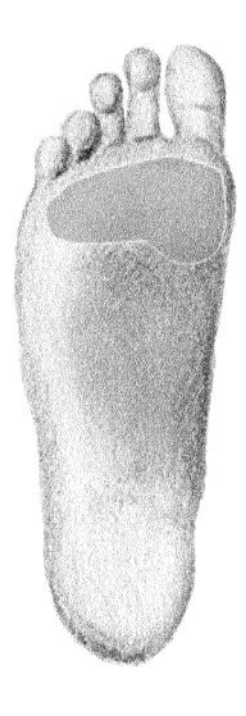

Kurcha

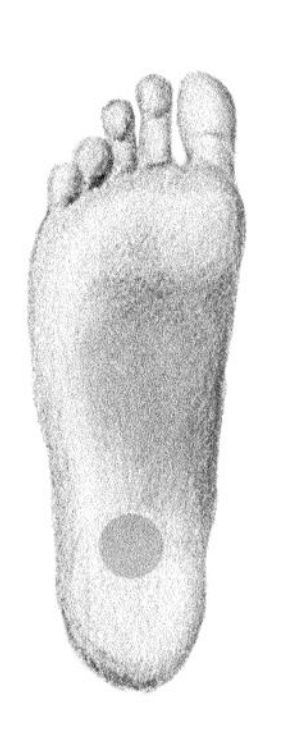

Kurchashira

### The thigh tendon Marma – Ani

The thigh tendon Marma (Ani) is equivalent to the Marma of the same name on the arms. The front point is about three to four fingers' width above the kneecap, with the back one directly opposite, above the back of the knee. Main applications include leg pain, fluid retention (oedema), poor circulation and kidney and pancreatic disease. Vata and Kapha dominate this Marma. The point on the muscle attachment of the extensor may be treated with the flat hand. Again support the Marma with your other hand, giving peace and comfort (see photo 1). This also applies to partner treatment. You can also massage with both thumbs (photos 2 and 3). Sedative, analgesic oils like joint soothe oil, for example, are very effective for muscle tension and leg pain or, for oedema, diuretic oils like juniper.

**Adhimarma:** Basti, Sushumna.

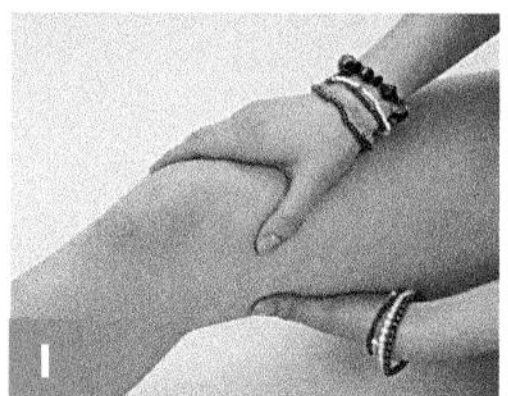

1

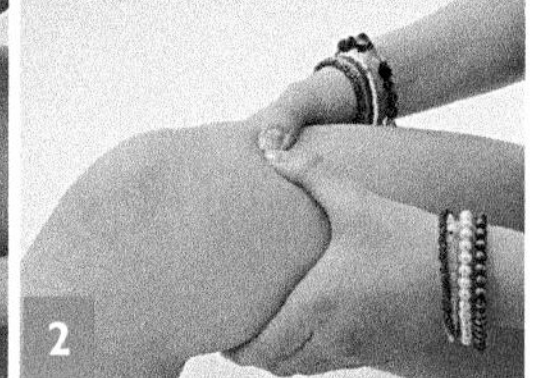

2

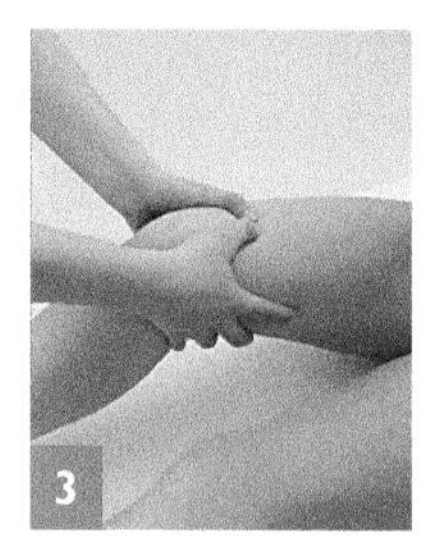

3

## The vessel Marma on the upper leg – Urvi

Like Ani Marma, Urvi controls water balance as well as circulation. As a vessel Marma it also brings heat, Agni, to the organs in the chest. Urvi is easy to find. Hold the middle of the thigh with one hand underneath, and the other above with your thumbs to the inside (photo 1). If you feel a little deeper through the muscle then you may feel the pulsing of the leg artery. The main point of the Marma is precisely here. The counterpoint is exactly opposite on the outside of the thigh.

Be very careful and delicate during treatment, preferably using the flat hand (photo 2); use the 1–3–5–7 treatment format, repeated several times. Please do not treat with pressure; it is not about massaging the blood vessels or muscles. We want to gently feel and enliven the field of consciousness of Urvi.

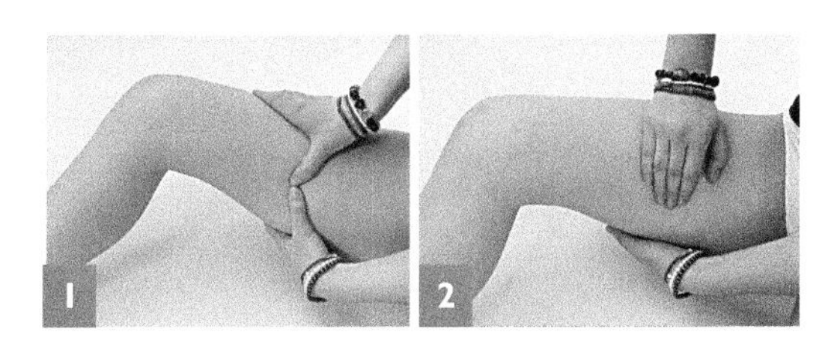

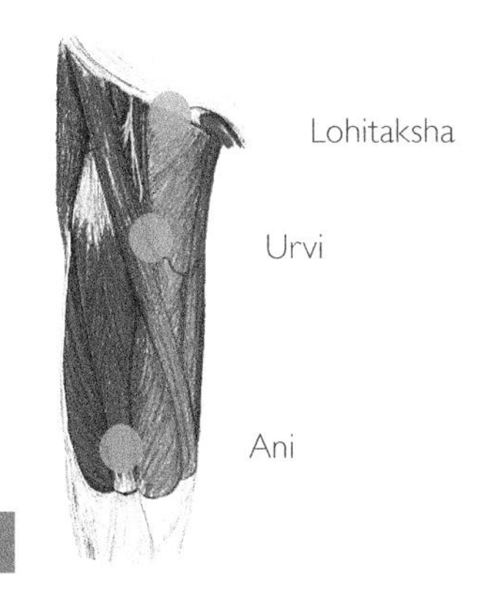


## The groin Marma – Lohitaksha

This vessel Marma lies in the groin, its centre about two finger-widths to the side of the pubic bone, where you can feel the leg artery pulsing. Its energy field extends over a larger area, going over the front of the hip region to the sides of the lower abdomen. As a vessel Marma it again regulates the blood vessels, nerves and lymphatic vessels that pass through. It is a very sensitive point that should only be treated with experience. Use a gentle up-and-down massage along the groin, the whole sideward pelvis and its organs: the colon, ovaries and lymphatic flow, as well as the hip joint and surrounding muscles, become relaxed. This treatment also promotes blood circulation. Even hip pain can be alleviated, especially if you use an analgesic, circulation-increasing oil such as joint soothe oil. The draining, downward movement stimulates and supports Apana Vata, which controls excretion.

## The pubic bone Marma – Vitapa

This corresponds to the Kakshadhara Marma at the shoulder. It is a finger-width laterally from the pubic bone, with its centre at the external opening of the inguinal canal, through which the spermatic cord passes in males. It controls the reproductive organs and menstruation and activates excretion processes (Apana Vata). Without medical experience, this Marma, like Lohitaksha, is too sensitive for partner treatment. However, gentle up-and-down massage in the groin area is fine for self-treatment. Lohitaksha and Vitapa are treated simultaneously in this way.

# The Seven Mahamarmas and Marmas of the Chest

On the front of the body we find the major Marmas, which are the centres of energy control in the organism. They control the seven Chakras and the basic, essential functions: the excretion, reproduction, digestion and distribution of all the substances that are essential for life, metabolism, emotions, intellect and perception.

The root Marma is Guda, which is located at the anus and pelvic floor. Its consciousness is earth-related, existential and reproduction-oriented, and it controls the large intestine and its excretions. It is the source of Shakti, creative energy, and in Vedic mythology is seen as a symbol of one of the three forms of expression of Mother Nature (Durga).

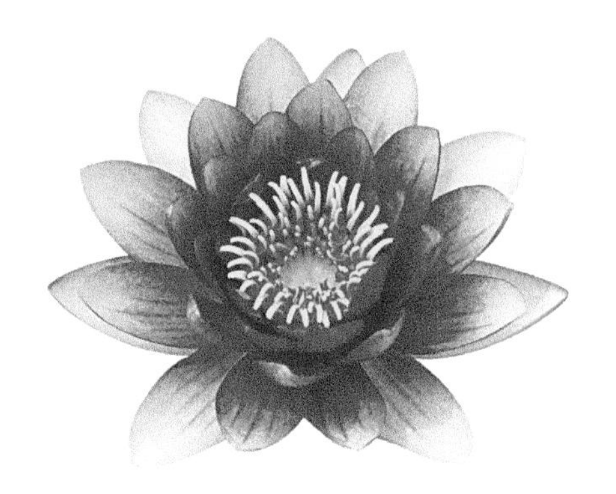

The bladder Marma (Basti) is the centre of energetic control of the pelvic organs, of sexual energy and excretion, especially of fluids.

In the navel Marma (Nabhi) we find the main energy of transformation for physical and mental digestion. It is a central point of the body, a Brahmasthan.

The heart Marma (Hridaya) is the main seat of sensitivity, of emotions and of life, the source of Ojas and also the main control centre for the distribution all vital substances. In the chest area we find further important Marmas, which are controlled by the heart Marma (Hridaya) and support its functions, principally in relation to the organs of the chest. According to Vedic mythology, the second expression of Mother Nature, Lakshmi, the goddess of fortune and the nourishing power of nature, wealth and health, dwells in the heart.

The three other major Marmas, Nila/Manya, Sthapani and Adhipati on the neck and head, are discussed in detail, starting on page 90. Saraswati, the third personification of Mother Nature, has her seat in the head or brain.

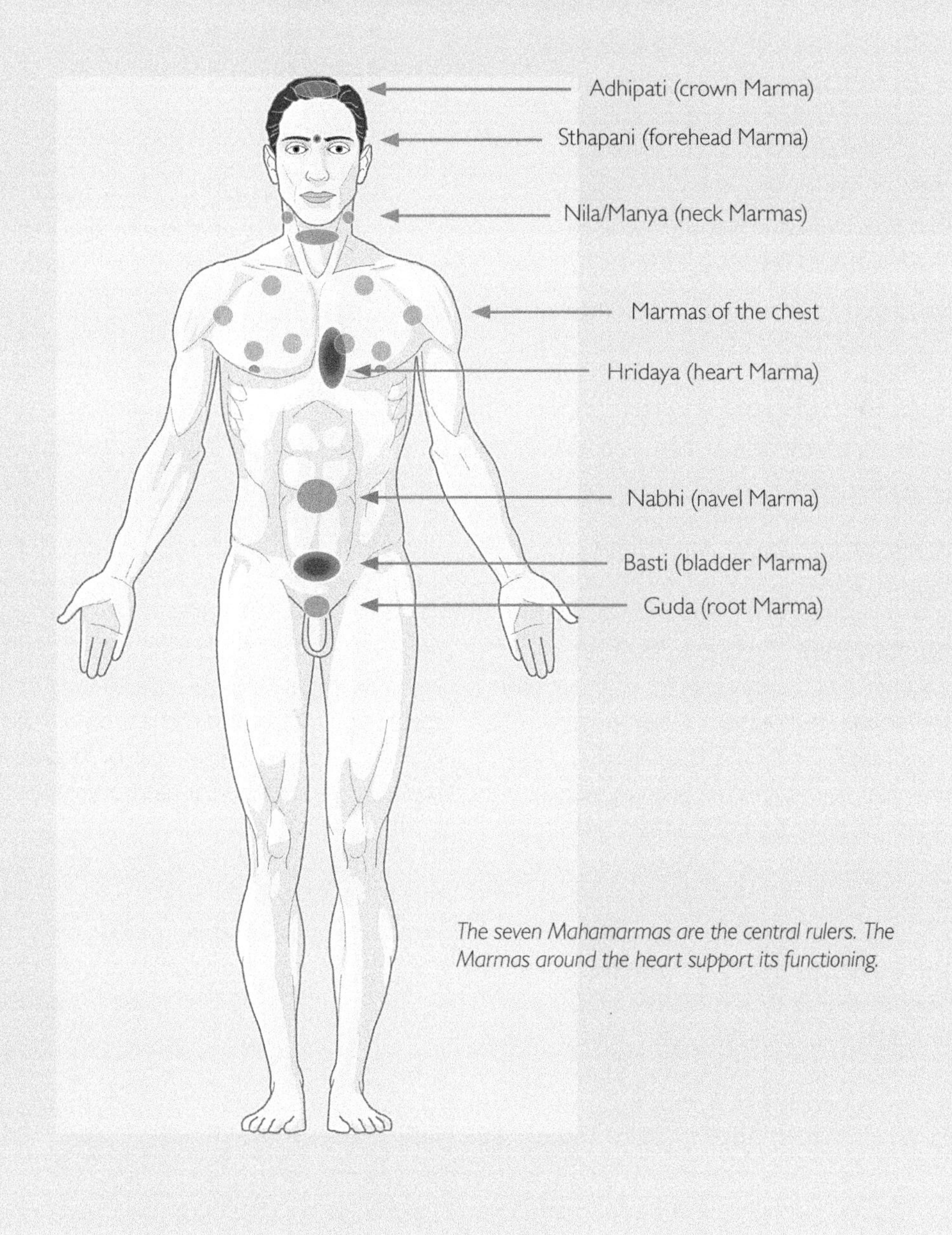


*The seven Mahamarmas are the central rulers. The Marmas around the heart support its functioning.*

## The pelvic floor Marma – Guda

Guda means 'anus', but also 'firewood', 'fire' and 'light'. It is the first of the major Marmas in the body centre, a large muscle Marma. Its centre is the anus and the rectum, but the whole area of the pelvic floor is within its aura.

**Application: Sexual disorders, diseases of the sex organs, sexual weakness and impotence, menstrual disorders, prostate diseases, haemorrhoids, elimination disorders of the urinary tract and colon, constipation, nervous weakness, fear of failure, existential fear.**

**Significance:** Guda is the energetic root of our being. Here we are existentially connected with the earth and also with the material security that we desire and need to get through life safely. Of the large central Marmas, Guda has a feminine, maternal nature, while Adhipati, the seventh and highest Marma, has a masculine, paternal nature. Guda is the source of Shakti, the creative, cosmic energy.

**Control function:** The pelvic floor Marma controls the first Chakra and is (as is the bladder Marma) involved in the control of excretory functions (Apana Vata). Its focus and energetic centre is in the large intestine; its main element is earth. In contrast, the bladder Marma dominates the water element and controls fluid excretion. Like the bladder Marma, Guda stores sexual energy and controls the function of the reproductive organs. Pelvic floor exercises have a direct effect on the muscle Marma Guda and strengthen it.

**Immediate effect:** Heat and energy in the pelvic floor area.

**How to find Guda:** The Marma is located at the anus and the pelvic floor. It extends into the rectum. The Marma is treated in Ayurveda primarily through various enemas, called Bastis. For Marma massage, the reference point for Guda is preferable. It lies over the tailbone.

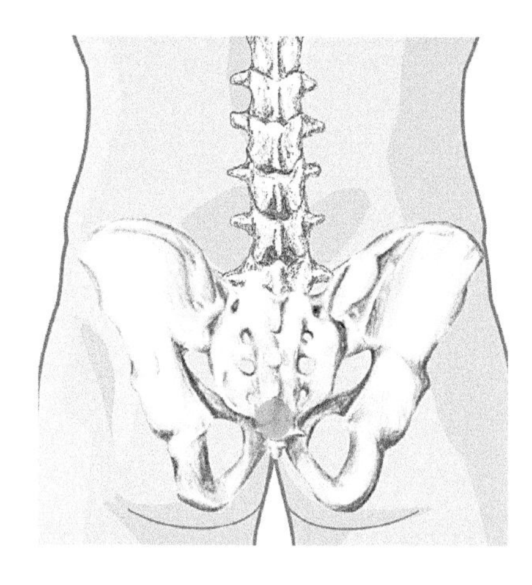

*Marmas of the lower back*

### OVERVIEW

**Marma type:** Mamsa (muscle Marma)

**1 point:** palm-sized area

**Peripheral Marma:** Kurchashira

**Effects:** controls the first Chakra, the excretion processes (Apana Vata), reproduction and the reproductive organs, Vata in the colon

**Oils:** dashamoola oil, Vata massage oil, sweet almond, lotus, sesame oil (in case of stress, nervous exhaustion or excess Vata); jasmine, rose or sandalwood oil (for cooling and for inflammations and excess Pitta)

**Adhimarma:** Guda

## Self-treatment

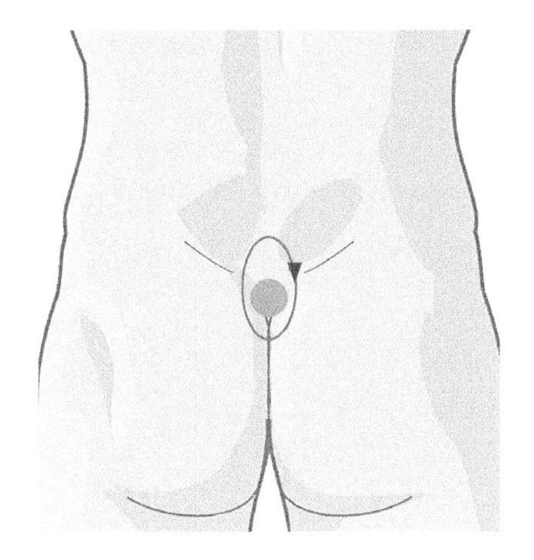

**Circular massage with the three fingers of the right hand:** The reference point of the Marma has its centre over the coccyx and its energetic expansion over the lower portion of the sacrum; this is easily accessible in self-treatment.

Sit comfortably and erect. Support the Marma energetically in its counterpoint by putting the left hand on the pubic bone. Place your right hand with the fingers on the sacrum. Gently perform circular massage movements with your index, middle and ring fingers. Repeat several times.

**Treatment time:** 1–3 minutes.

## Partner treatment

The partner treatment is similar to self-treatment but is best performed as part of the whole lower back treatment (pages 82–83).

**Contact:** The right hand rests on the sacrum. The left hand is placed a hand's breadth away from the pubic bone if your partner is sitting up, and above the top of the head if your partner is lying down.

## The bladder Marma – Basti

Basti means 'bladder', but also 'home'. It is the seat of government of the large tendon Marma of the bladder.

**Application: Bladder diseases, irritable bladder, exhaustion and nervous disorders, menstrual disorders, sexual disorders, gynaecological problems, prostate problems, flatulence, colon problems, back pain, hip pain.**

**Significance:** The bladder is the seat of the lowest of the three main Marmas. Instinctive consciousness with its earthly feelings and sexual needs manifests in the bladder Marma. If it is healthy, it gives basic trust; we can let ourselves go and feel grounded and secure.

**Control function:** The bladder Marma controls the second Chakra, excretion (Apana Vata), especially of the urinary organs but also of the colon, and menstruation. It stores sexual energy and controls the function of the sex organs. As one of the three main Marmas it is responsible for a wide range of physical functions. The main energy channel springing from it, the bladder meridian, starts on the inner corners of the right and left eye and runs as a pair over the frontal sinuses, skull, neck, back and legs to the outer side of the little toes. It also monitors muscles and body fat.

**Immediate effect:** Relaxation in the lower abdomen, calming of the mind, reduced tension in the lower back, general reassurance.

**How to find Basti:** The Marma is exactly over the bladder, just above the pubic bone. It is about the size of a palm, which is about the size of the urinary bladder. In its centre is the Bindu, containing the highest concentration of Prana.

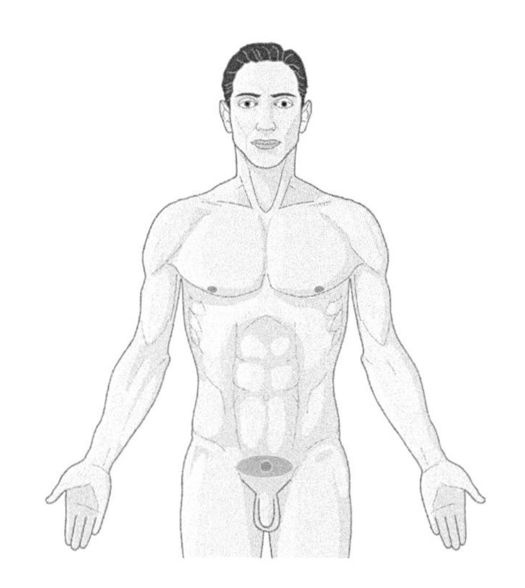

### OVERVIEW

**Marma type:** Snayu (tendon Marma)

**I point:** palm-sized area

**Peripheral Marma:** Indrabasti

**Effect:** controls the second Chakra, the excretion processes (Apana Vata), muscle and fat tissue, the sex organs, reproduction, Vata in the colon

**Oils:** dashamoola oil, Vata massage oil, almond, lotus, sesame oil (for stress, nervous fatigue, irritable bladder, excess Vata); jasmine, rose or sandalwood oil (cooling, for inflammation, excess Pitta)

**Adhimarma:** Basti

## Self-treatment

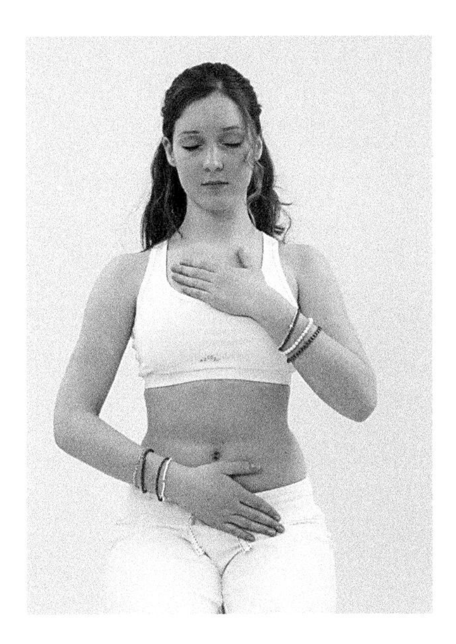

**Circular massage with the palm of the hand:** You can sit up or lie down. This Marma treatment is very soothing with or without oil and has a balancing effect on the lower abdomen, pelvic organs and your entire physical and mental condition. Place your left hand on the heart Marma and with your right hand massage over the Basti area slowly and gently in a clockwise circle (see illustration). Repeat the 1–3–5–7 treatment format 2 to 3 times.

**Treatment time:** 3–5 minutes.

## Partner treatment

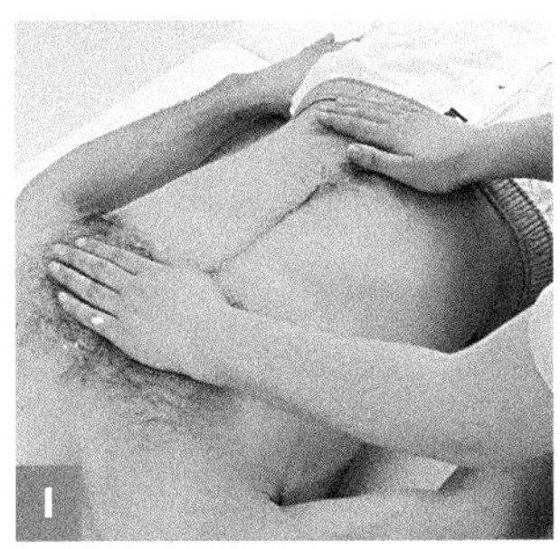


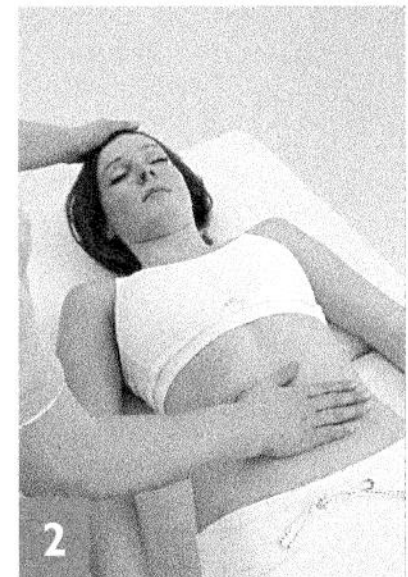


Partner treatment is done in the same way as self-treatment. Sit to the right of your partner so that you feel relaxed and comfortable and the treatment is comfortable for you.

**Contact:** First place your left hand over the forehead, with the right one over the bladder. Then the left hand moves over the heart, while the right remains over the bladder (photo 1).

**Resting the hand on the Marma:** If you are treating without oil, you could simply place your right hand on the bladder Marma while the left rests on the crown of the head (if your partner feels this is comfortable) (photo 2). Heat and Prana from your hand will have a soothing and healing influence on the bladder Marma.

## The navel Marma – Nabhi

Nabhi is a big blood vessel Marma around the navel, which is the centre of this Marma.

**Application: Indigestion, abdominal cramp, restlessness, anxiety, intestinal inflammation, Crohn's disease, ulcerative colitis, flatulence, loss of balance in life.**

**Significance:** The navel is the centre of the body, a Brahmasthan in the language of Ayurveda. It is the absolute point of rest and the source of order and health. If the navel Marma is in harmony, we are at home in our body and feel centred. As beings in the wombs of our mothers, we are nourished through the navel by our mother's placenta. The navel maintains this nourishing function throughout our life, but after birth in an energetic way. The navel Marma is regarded as a Prana centre from which, according to the Vedic texts, emerge all the 72,000 energy channels, which are the meridians or Nadis. In the navel Marma we touch the root of our existence.

**Control function:** Nabhi controls the third Chakra, Manipura. When the Chakra is in harmony, this wheel spins in a clockwise direction. Its main task is to ensure the flow of nutrients along the various digestive stages from the stomach through the small intestine and large intestine towards the rectum. The fire at the centre of our life, the digestive fire, Agni, also resides here and is raised by the wind of Samana Vata and regulated by the navel Marma.

**Immediate effect:** Increase of peace and strength in the abdominal region, mental calmness, relaxation in the abdomen, a feeling of warmth around the navel, gurgling noises resulting from the dissolution of intestinal cramps.

**How to find Nabhi:** The navel is the centre of the Marma, which extends about a hand's breadth.

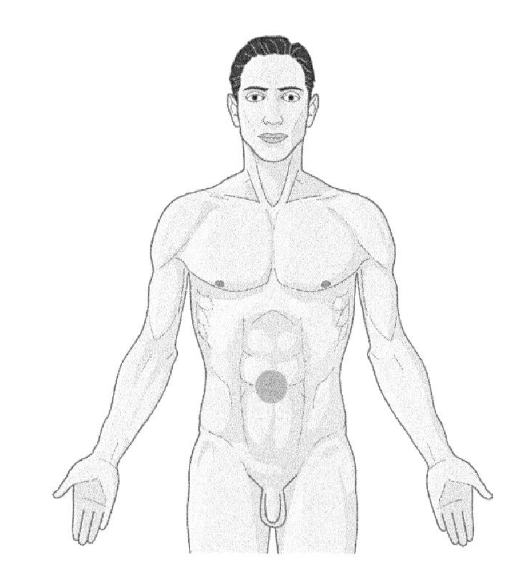

### OVERVIEW

**Marma type:** Sira (vessel Marma)

**I point:** an area the size of the hand

**Peripheral Marma:** Talahridaya

**Effect:** controls the navel Chakra, the Vishvodhara energy channel (page 81), the digestive system (Pachaka, Samana Vata, Agni), the distribution of nutrients via the bloodstream and the channels of the nutrient flow (Vyana Vata), liver, bile and pancreas (Ranjaka) and Pitta Dosha in general

**Oils:** Vata massage oil, fennel, almond and sesame oil (for stress, abdominal cramps, excess Vata); jasmine, rose or sandalwood oil (cooling, for inflammation, excess Pitta)

**Adhimarma:** Nabhi

## Self-treatment

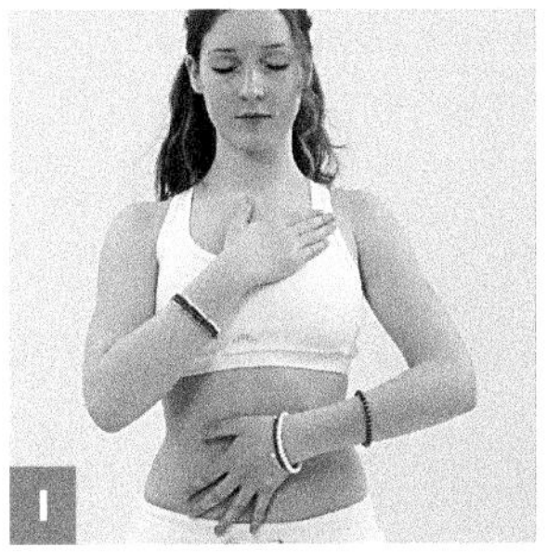

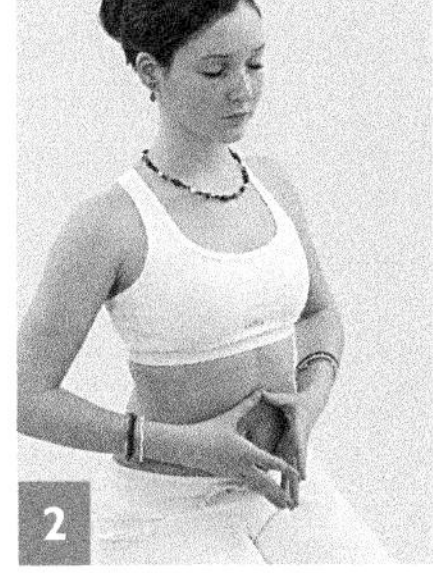

**Circular massage with the palm of the hand:** With or without oil, sitting up or lying down, this Marma treatment has an extremely soothing and balancing effect on the whole abdominal area and your entire physical and mental condition.

Place your left hand on the heart Marma and with your right hand massage the stomach in a clockwise direction using very gentle, slow movements over a large area. The hand and fingers are flat; the navel is the centre. Massage gently with no pressure; use only the weight of the hand. Repeat the 1–3–5–7 format 2 to 4 times.

**Circular massage on the navel:** For a more profound effect, circular massage on the navel itself is recommended. Apply a little oil around the navel and on the navel itself, and massage it very gently, in a slow, calm manner, starting with the tip of the middle finger on the navel. Repeat the standard treatment format 2 to 4 times.

**Mudras on the navel:** To finish, place your hand on your stomach with the centre of the palm over the navel and the little finger pointing down to the bladder (photo 1 – this Mudra should be performed with the left hand). One of the best Mudras for the navel Marma is Hakini (photo 2). With or without preparatory massage, this strengthens the whole abdominal region, bringing warmth and calmness, strengthens the centre of life, and brings confidence and peace. The thumbs and little fingers rest on the belly, forming a circle, with the navel at the centre.

**Treatment time:** 3–5 minutes.

## Partner treatment

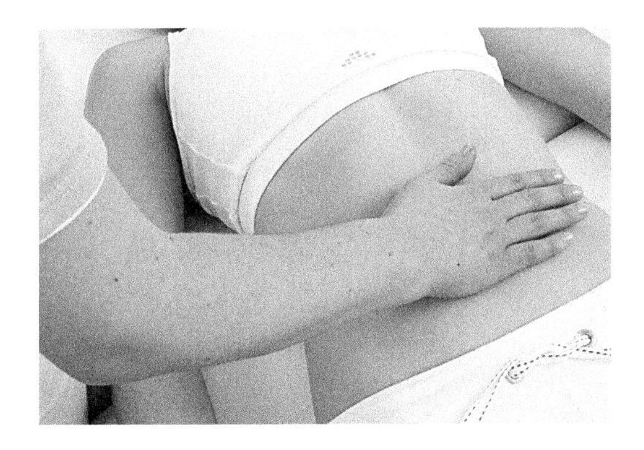

This does not differ significantly from the self-treatment. In the second option, where we are only treating the navel itself, instead of using the middle finger, massage the navel with the tip of your thumb. Sit on the right of your partner, so that you remain relaxed and the treatment is comfortable for you.

**Contact:** First the left hand is placed over the heart, with the right one over the navel. In the next step the right hand moves over the bladder Marma, with the left over the navel. Finally we also connect the head Marmas with the navel: the left hand over the forehead or crown of the head and the right again over the bladder.

## The great heart Marma – Hridaya

The heart is seen in Ayurveda as the seat of the soul (Atma) and, for this reason, Hridaya is the most important of all the Marmas. Connections emerge from Hridaya to all the other Marmas. It is a vessel Marma.

**Application: Nervous heart complaints, sorrow, strengthening of self-confidence, supportive treatment for organic and vegetative heart disorders, circulatory disorders, stress-related high blood pressure, spinal weakness and discomfort, chest disease, diseases of the lungs and bronchial infections. Has health benefits for the entire organism; is involved in the formation of breast milk.**

**Significance:** The harmonization of Hridaya bestows inner peace and opens the heart for love and compassion, but also strengthens courage, confidence, warmth and cordiality, humour, inner happiness and emotional intelligence.

**Control function:** The heart Marma controls all the energy pathways and Marmas of the organism, the great blood vessels that supply the respiratory system and the lymphatic system, and the channels that distribute the first essence of food (Rasa). The heart is the main seat of Ojas, the basis of immunity, happiness, health and joy of life. Its Marma controls the fourth Chakra and is the seat of emotional intelligence (Sadhaka Pitta).

**Immediate effect:** The treatment deepens breathing, calms the heart and simultaneously has a warming effect on the solar plexus. Also Brihati, the Marma on the opposite side, is calmed and strengthened by the treatment of Hridaya. Brihati is, figuratively speaking, the male partner of the heart, watching its back and supporting it in all issues. It, too, is a vessel Marma.

**How to find Hridaya:** The Marma is above the breastbone and slightly to the left (see diagram below) and is about the size of a hand. If you go up and down with the ball of a flat, opened hand along the breastbone, you feel an increased sensitivity in the area of Hridaya.

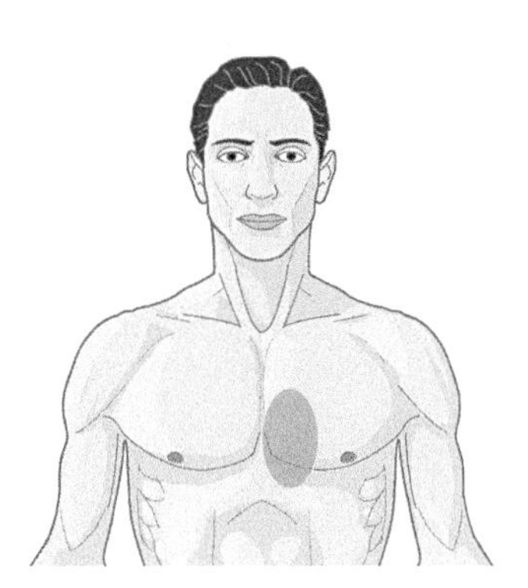

### OVERVIEW

**Marma type:** Sira (vessel Marma)

**I point:** central Marma, over the breastbone

**Supporting Marma:** Brihati

**Peripheral Marma:** Talahridaya

**Effects:** harmonizes all other Marmas, gives peace, strengthens self-confidence and emotional intelligence. Increases Ojas, strengthens Prana (mind power and intelligence), Sadhaka (satisfaction and inner happiness), Vyana (circulation), Tarpaka (nervous system), Avalambaka (strength of the back), Varuna Nadi and the fourth Chakra (Anahata) (see diagram on page 81).

**Oils:** Vata massage oil, Vata aroma oil, sweet almond oil (to calm Vata); sandalwood, lotus, Worry Free, Even Temper, jasmine, rose (emotionally balancing)

**Adhimarma:** Hridaya

## Self-treatment

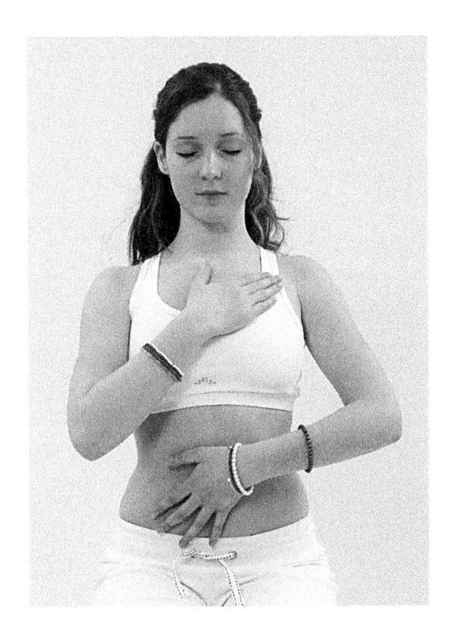

Sit comfortably and upright. Soothingly place the left hand with its centre (Talahridaya) on the navel. The little finger points vertically down towards the bladder. Place the right hand over the breastbone, as shown in the picture above. With the palm and ball of the hand, with fingers slightly stretched, circle clockwise gently and very softly, starting at the bottom right and ending at the bottom left. Move your hand in a natural rhythm with the breath. Repeat the standard treatment format 2 to 4 times.

**Finishing the treatment:** Place the right hand on the heart Marma and the left hand on the navel.

**Mudras:** The treatment of the heart Marma can be effectively complemented by Mudras: Anjali Mudra (meditation, devotion; page 111) and the Mudra for self-confidence (page 118).

**Treatment time:** 3–5 minutes.

## Partner treatment

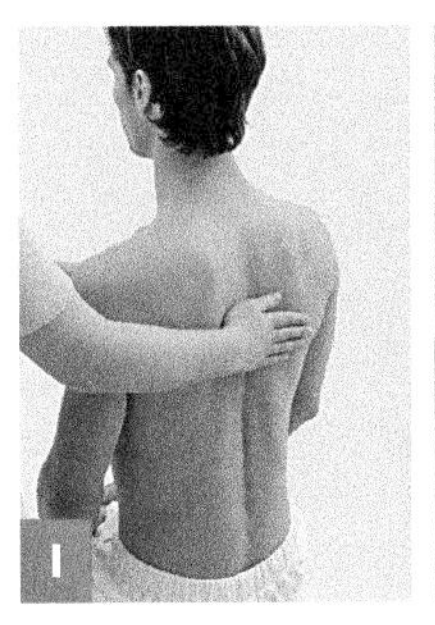

1

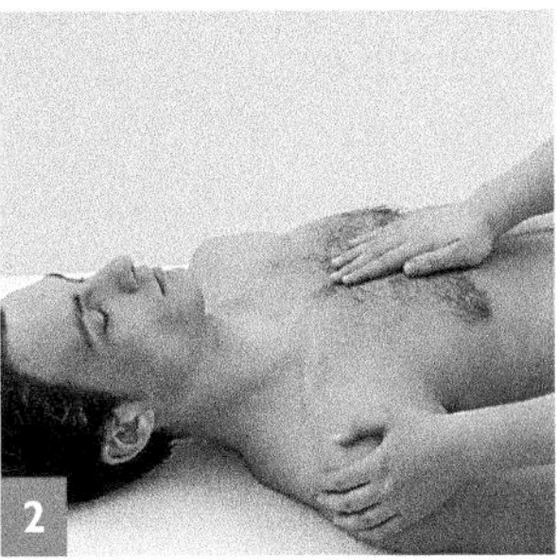

2

**Contact:** If your partner is lying down, stand to the right of your partner; your left hand rests over the heart, with the right over the bladder Marma. Then place the right hand over the heart and the left over the forehead.

If your partner is sitting, stand to the left and place the left hand over the heart and the right hand over Brihati.

**Treatment:** Your partner is either lying down or sitting upright and relaxed. If they are sitting, then place your left hand on their back, opposite the heart, which is Brihati Marma (photo 1). Now do very slow, gentle, oval movements over the heart Marma in a clockwise direction with the ball of the right hand. Your movements should be in tune with the breath of your partner – upwards when they breathe in, and downwards when they breathe out.

If your partner is lying down then stand to their right. Treat the Marma with your right hand (photo 2) in the same way as described for self-treatment.

## Additional Marmas in the chest area

The great heart Marma is the absolute ruler in the entire chest region and the following points belong to its immediate territory and support it. The Marmas in the immediate vicinity are directly affected by treatment of Hridaya but all the other Marmas in the chest area are also affected because of the increased flow of Prana and Ojas. They benefit directly from treatment of Hridaya. However, we can also include them in a more comprehensive therapy by treating all the points of the front and lateral chest area. On page 136 we introduce this therapy together with other Ayurvedic treatments.

Three of these four Marmas surrounding the heart are also vessel Marmas; only Stanarohita, the Marma field of vital energy of the two chest muscles, is a muscle Marma. The front chest Marmas strengthen the thoracic organs and the immune and nervous systems, and they support the cardiovascular system.

The 1–3–5–7 treatment format applies to all these Marmas, or just follow your feelings and sense of well-being. But for all chest Marmas it is important that you have time and peace for feeling into the treatment.

### The root of the chest – Stanamula

This vessel Marma has the nipple as the centre of its energy but also includes other points around the breast. In the context of Ayurvedic massage, the nipple is usually included in massage of the breast. Since it is very sensitive, for Marma treatment we recommend massaging the breast area with both hands, simultaneously using circular movements in opposite directions. This treatment includes the chest muscle Marma, Stanarohita.

### The chest muscle Marma – Stanarohita

Stanarohita includes the pectoral muscle, the mammary glands and the surrounding tissues. Its centre is to the left and right of the sternum on the origin of the pectoralis major muscle approximately two finger-widths above the line between the nipples. As a muscle Marma it stores power and energy. It also has great influence on the nervous system, respiratory system and Prana, the circulation (Vyana Vata), the lungs and, of course, the formation of breast milk. The treatment that we described for Stanamula (above) includes Stanarohita. Gentle self-treatment of the female breast tightens it, has a general strengthening effect, strengthens the breast muscles, the nervous system and lungs, and promotes formation of breast milk.

## The Marma of the armpit – Apalapa

Apalapa is also a vessel Marma, and sits in the armpit just below Lohitaksha and the muscle attachment of the small chest muscle (M. pectoralis minor). It is very sensitive, and treatment is only suitable in the context of medical indications – for example, for treatment of paralysis or shoulder problems. A gentle, sensitive self-treatment with the three fingers of one hand is useful in mild shoulder or arm discomfort, in circulatory disorders of the arm and hand and in nervous heart complaints.

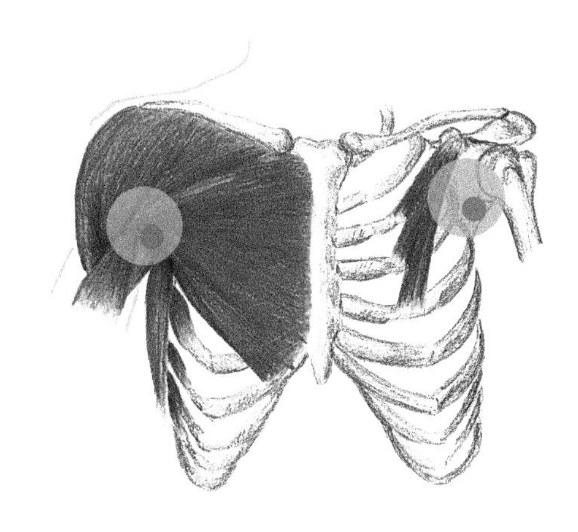

*Location of Apalapa*

## The vessel Marma of the chest – Apastambha

Apastambha is situated above the point where the two main bronchi divide and the pulmonary arteries have their source. The two main points lie in the space between the second and third rib on the left and right of the sternum. Its effect extends into the upper abdomen, especially the stomach, where it supports the formation of gastric mucus (Kledaka Kapha). Some Ayurvedic sources say that it also controls the formation of fat and bone tissue and their transport channels. When you put your flat hand on both points, you may also feel that emotions belonging to the heart, and also to the stomach or solar plexus, are stored here. The complete treatment, including all chest Marmas, can be found on pages 136–137.

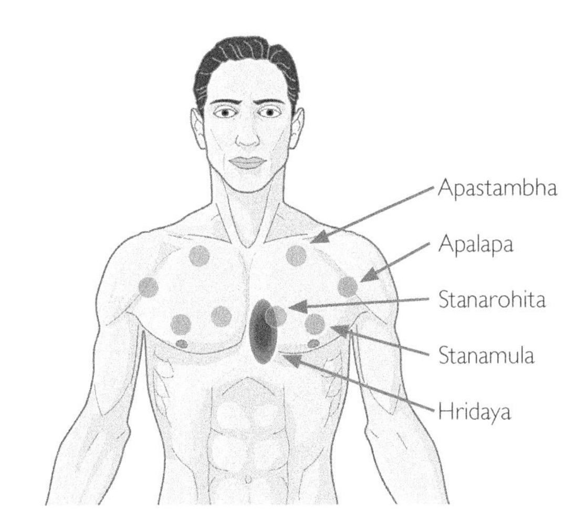


*The Marmas of the chest*

# Marmas of the Pelvis and Back

While the front of the body is covered with Marmas which are busy receiving and absorbing energies and which are very sensitive and vulnerable, the Marmas on the back shield and provide protection. It is not surprising, therefore, that six of the eight bone Marmas are found on the back of the body. Only the two temple Marmas, Shanka, lie on the head, facing sidewards. The bone Marmas protect vulnerable soft parts and organs of the body: the intestines and organs in the pelvis and chest. The Shankas protect the highly sensitive area of the temple and the underlying parts of the brain.

The spine also carries energy directed upwards and is the most important and principal pillar for the flow of Prana. The three main energy channels run along the spine with *Sushumna* in the centre, *Ida* to the left and *Pingala* on the right. First they supply the central Marmas and the seven Chakras which are connected to them (see figure opposite). From here thousands of Nadis or meridians, distributed all over the body, connect all the Marmas in a complex network. Ida and Pingala proceed to the brain and go from there to the third eye, Sthapani Marma, and thence to the nose, eyes and ears. We will elaborate on this in the section on head Marmas (page 90).

In Sukshma Marma treatment we encourage the flow of Prana in Ida, Pingala and Sushumna to nourish all the organs along the spine that are connected to the Marmas and Chakras.

The back Marmas are difficult to reach in self-treatment and are therefore particularly suitable when working with a partner. The complete back treatment, as described from page 134, is very effective in that it includes all the Marmas of the pelvis, back and shoulders.

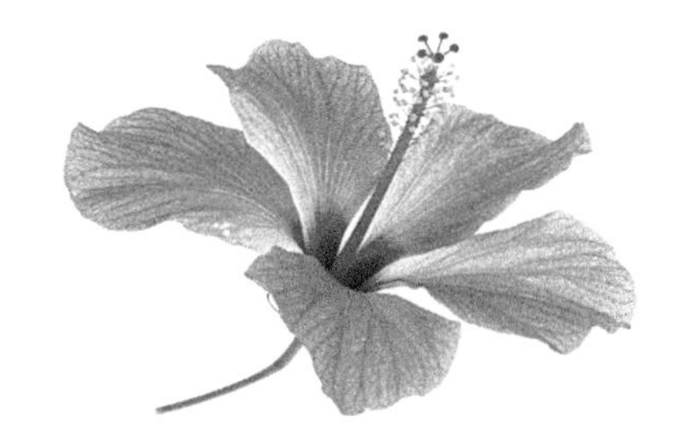

## RELATIONSHIP OF THE SIX NADIS AND THE SEVEN CHAKRAS

**6. Sushumna Nadi**
Marma: Sthapani, Adhipati
*Opening: Third eye, eyes*

**5. Saraswati Nadi**
Marma: Tip of the tongue, the centre of the dip below the lower lip
*Opening: Mouth, pharynx*

**4. Varuna Nadi**
Marma: Hridaya
*Opening: Skin*

**3. Vishvodhara Nadi**
Marma: Nabhi
*Opening: Navel*

**2. Kuhu Nadi**
Marma: Basti
*Opening: Penis, vagina*

**1. Alambusha Nadi**
Marma: Guda
*Opening: Anus*

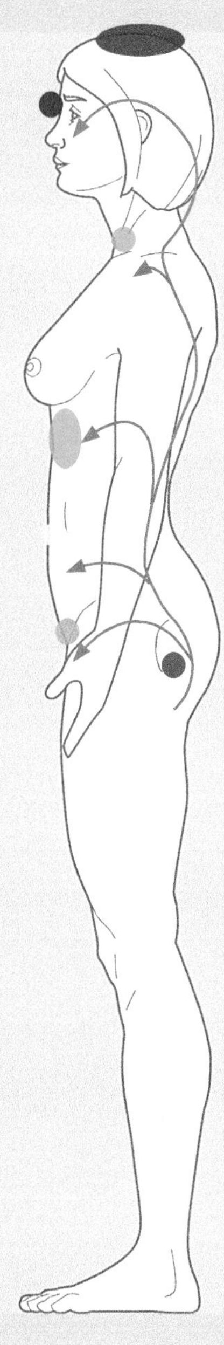

**7. Sahasrara Chakra**

**6. Ajna Chakra**

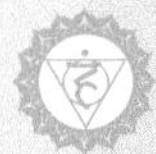
**5. Vishuddha Chakra**

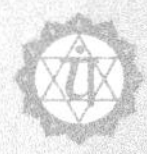
**4. Anahata Chakra**

**3. Manipura Chakra**

**2. Svadisthana Chakra**

**1. Muladhara Chakra**

*Subtle energy channels originating at the base of the spine supply the Chakras and Marmas with Pranic energy.*

## The Marmas of the pelvis along the lumbar spine

We are going to discuss the Marmas of the lower back and pelvis together because they interact very closely and are generally treated together. They form the basis for strength in the pelvis and lumbar spine which hold the body straight and upright. This is also the main seat of an important Subdosha of Kapha: Avalambaka, the 'spine strengthener'. This gives stability and strength not only to the lumbar region but along the entire spine and chest and supports associated organs, especially the heart. The effective range of the Marmas of the lower back and pelvis extends to the hips and the organs in the pelvis. The hips are important areas where Kapha (i.e. power and energy) accumulates and where connections to the lymphatic system can be found.

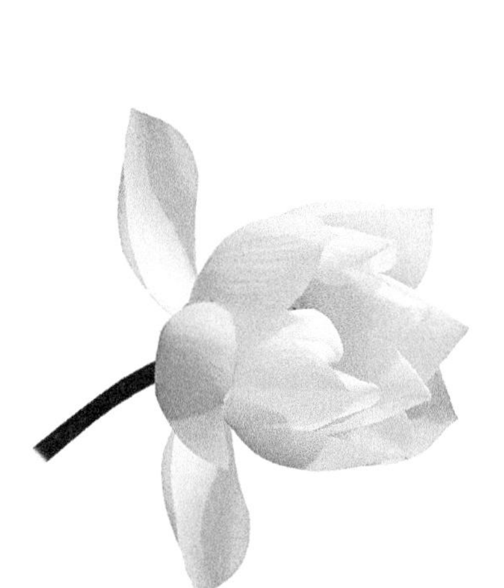

### Kukundara – the sacroiliac joint Marma

The two central points of this joint Marma sit on the two hip dimples (spina iliaca posterior superior) which are often clearly visible above the buttocks. If there is a blockage in the sacroiliac joint, the point on the blocked side can be painful, and this pain often radiates to the hip and down along the back of the leg, imitating sciatic pain. The surrounding muscles can then become tight and sensitive to pressure. This Marma is on the energy path of the bladder and controls the pelvic organs, especially the bladder, ovaries, uterus, small intestine and large intestine, and the excretion processes (Apana Vata). The second Chakra Svadisthana communicates with this Marma.

### Katikataruna – that which comes from the hip

The connecting point of this bone Marma is located in the centre of the buttock muscle and on an imaginary line between the ischium (seat bone) and the trochanter of the hip bone. It controls the bone and skeletal system, the lubrication of the joints and the sweat glands. Gentle massage on this area mainly calms Vata in the pelvic area (Apana, Samana).

### Nitamba – the ilium bone Marma

The centre of this bone Marma is located in the top outer quarter of each buttock (see diagram below), and its energy field extends to the ilium and the sacrum as well as the joint between the two. It protects the pelvis and also controls the flow of the first essence of food (Rasa), the lymphatic system in the pelvis, body fat, the skeletal system and the kidneys. Nitamba is an important Vata and Kapha point. It is involved when the sacroiliac joint becomes blocked and the surrounding area is painful. Gentle Marma massage loosens the joint and relaxes the pelvis and leg.

### Parshvasandhi – the flank

The range of this blood vessel Marma extends from its main location right or left of the lowest lumbar vertebra from the sacrum up to the top of the 12th rib. It controls blood supply to the kidneys and is a stress Marma, being connected energetically with the adrenal glands which excrete stress hormones. Like Kukundara (see page 82), it also controls the second Chakra. The ovaries, the digestive system, excretion processes and respiratory airways belong to its sphere of influence. We can treat Parshvasandhi ourselves. When seated, we put our hands wide open on the flanks. The tips of the ring finger and little finger touch the lateral region of the fifth lumbar vertebra. The hands rest on the kidneys. Even putting the hands on the Marma soothes and strengthens it, and with gentle up-and-down strokes we relax and revive it (see page 136, back treatment).

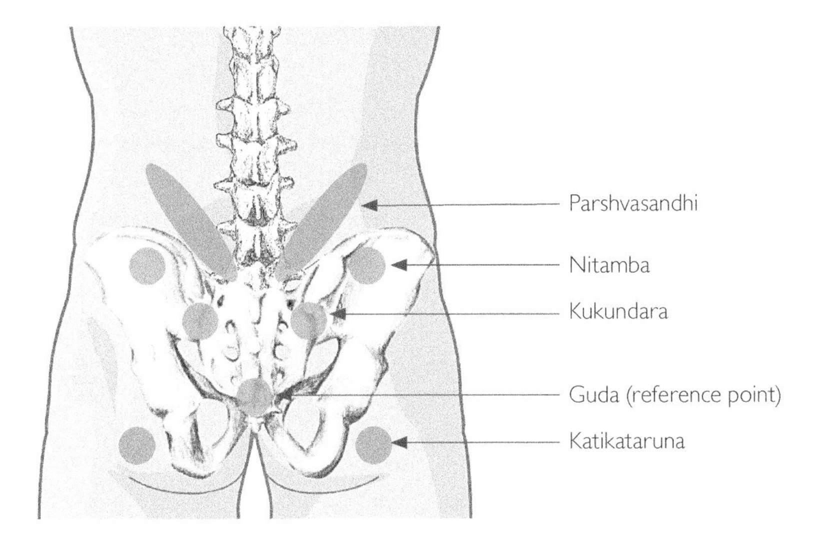


*Marmas of the lower back*

## The large Marma of the back – Brihati

Brihati means 'big, extended'. This is a large vessel Marma located between the shoulder blades, left and right of the spine.

**Application: Organic and psychological heart disease, heart failure, lung and bronchial disease, cough, sorrow, lack of confidence, discouragement, back pain, inner tension.**

**Significance:** Brihati is the seat of the consciousness of courage, strength and sincerity. Weakness of the mid-back occurs if the Marma is weakened; for example, if we experience grief, feel the burden of life as being too heavy or if we lack self-confidence. Brihati lies opposite the heart on the back. It is the mid-back strengthener, the Marma that 'strengthens the back' of the heart Marma. Heart Marma and Brihati act together like mother and father.

**Control function:** As a vessel Marma it guards over the flow of blood and lymph to the thoracic organs, the armpits and chest. Brihati encompasses several small Marmas which lie on the energy channel of the bladder (Basti Marma) and control the functioning of the lungs, heart, circulation and stomach. Brihati communicates with the third or navel Chakra (Manipura). This Marma is dominated by Kapha in the form of strength and power (Tarpaka, Avalambaka), Pitta as the Dosha of courage and Vata, which distributes energy (Vyana).

**Immediate effect:** Relaxation of the back, shoulders, arms and breathing.

**How to find Brihati:** The centre of the Marma lies between the shoulder blades, left and right of the spine. The whole Marma is larger and is about the length of a hand.

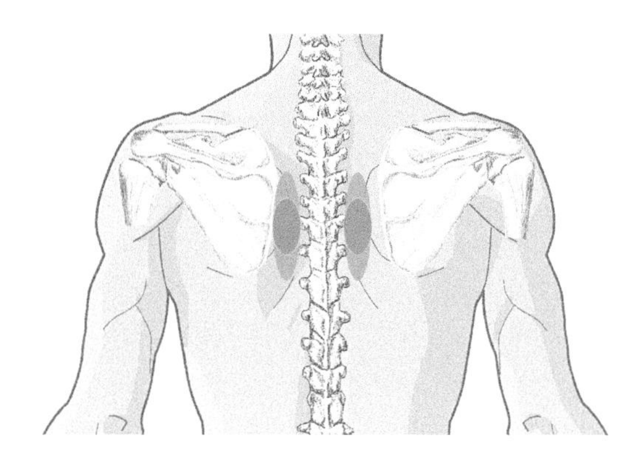

### OVERVIEW

**Marma type:** sira (vessel Marma)

**2 points:** 1 point to the left and 1 point to the right of the spinal column

**Peripheral Marma:** the opposite point of Talahridaya on the hands and feet

**Effects:** controls the navel Chakra, strengthens the back, heart and lungs (Avalambaka, Tarpaka), gives courage (Sadhaka); monitors circulation (Vyana), blood and lymph flow in the chest area and perspiration on the back

**Oils:** relaxing, invigorating and refreshing treatment oils such as MA 628 joint oil, sesame, almond, lemon, lemongrass, rose, rosewood, Brahmi

**Adhimarma:** Hridaya, Sushumna, Adiprana

## Self-treatment

The Marma is not accessible for direct self-treatment. It can be strengthened and harmonized with Yoga Asanas (see page 119). Both the prayer Mudra (page 111) and the Mudra for self-confidence (page 118) strengthen this Marma.

## Partner treatment

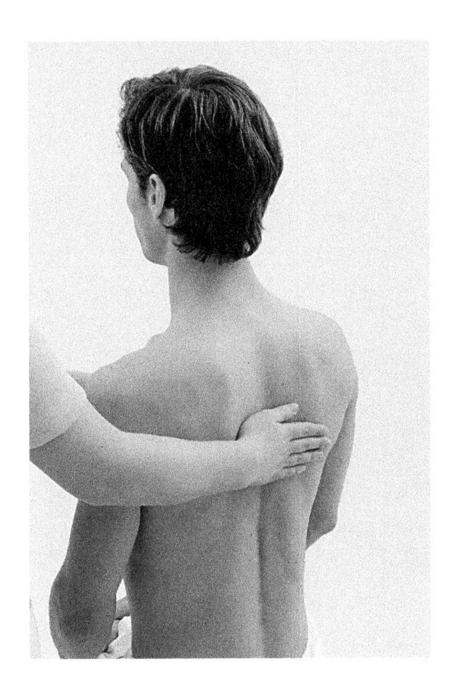

**Contact:** Stand to the left of your partner with your left hand resting over their heart, and the right over the back Marma.

**The hands strengthen courage and the Marma:** Your partner sits up straight and relaxed with closed eyes. You stand to the left. Your left hand is above the heart, with the right over the big back Marma (see illustration above). Give rest and strength for one or two minutes to the two Marmas, which work together as mother and father for the welfare of the body. This is similar to the treatment of the heart Marma (pages 76–77) but with the hands reversed.

**Massage with the palm of the hand:** While the left hand stays on the heart Marma, massage gently and calmly up and down along Brihati, keeping the hand horizontal. The fingers are touching and the whole hand is in contact with the back, with the palm moving up and down the spine. Repeat the treatment format several times.

**Treatment time:** 3–4 minutes.

## The Marma of the shoulder blade – Amsaphalaka

Amsaphalaka means 'shoulder blade'. This bone Marma covers a large area: the whole shoulder blade and the area near the spine. The main point is located on the upper inner shoulder blade angle, with the central point being exactly in the middle of the scapula.

**Application:** **Shoulder and arm pain, paralysis and numbness in the arm, indigestion.**

**Significance:** As with all bone Marmas, the shoulder blade offers protection. Heart, lungs and the large blood vessels in the chest are vital organs that the shoulder blade protects in case of attack or injury from behind. But psychological injuries can also be located here: we tend to lift the shoulder blades when danger threatens. Tension and anxiety are often found in this Marma.

**Control function:** The main point of the Marma is in the centre of the shoulder blade, and corresponds to the vital point of the small intestine meridian that crosses here. In addition to its energetic effect on the upper back, shoulders and arms, this Marma also monitors the airways (Pranavaha Shrotas), lungs, heart, the fourth Chakra, the cardiovascular system and the digestive fire.

**Immediate effect:** Relaxation of the back, shoulders, arms and breathing.

**How to find Amsaphalaka:** The centre of the Marma lies in the middle of the shoulder blade. This point is about the size of the tip of the thumb and is a bit painful to pressure. The whole shoulder blade is also in the energy field of the Marma, and the muscle attachments on the inner and upper edge of the shoulder blade are effective treatment areas.

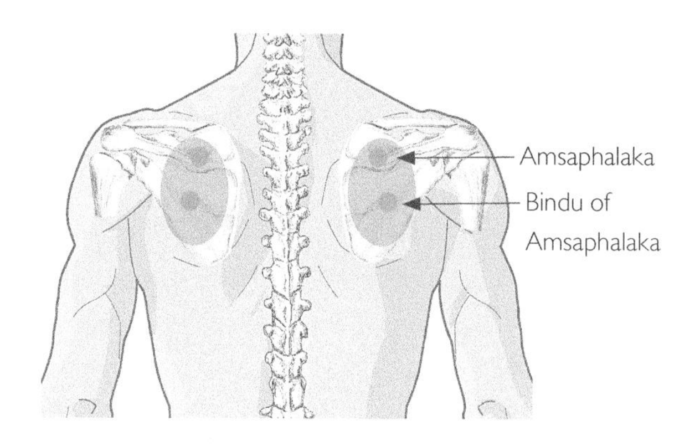


### OVERVIEW

**Marma type:** Asthi (bone Marma)

**2 points:** 1 point on each shoulder blade

**Peripheral Marma:** back of the thumb, distal phalanx

**Effects:** monitors the heart, lungs, airways, Udana Vata, Prana Vata, small intestine (Pachaka)

**Oil:** Vata massage oil with Vata essential oil, sesame, almond, lavender, jasmine, Brahmi (relaxing)

**Adhimarma:** Nabhi, Hridaya, Udana, Adiprana, Sushumna, Emotional Relief

## Self-treatment

The point is not accessible to direct self-treatment. Through Yoga Asanas (from page 119), however, it can be energetically harmonized.

## Partner treatment

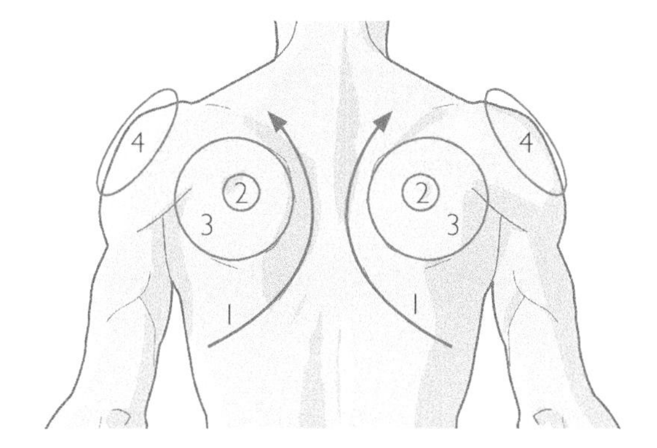


*Sequence and strokes for upper back and shoulders*

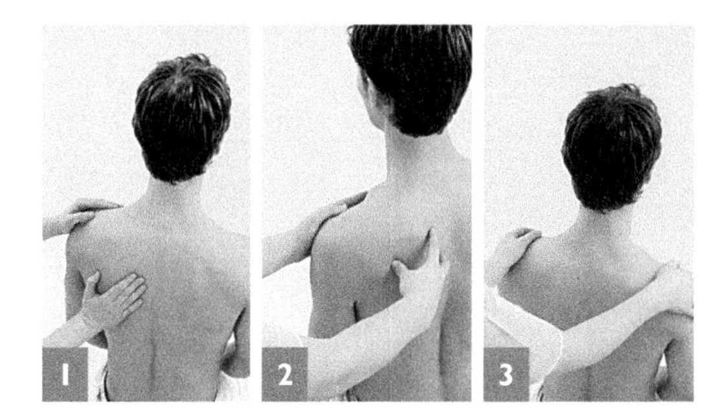


**Contact:** The left hand is over the heart, with the right over the left shoulder blade.

**Moon massage around the shoulder blade:** Your partner sits upright and relaxed. Hold their left shoulder from the outside and front with your left hand, while the right hand massages up and down in a moon shape along the inner angle of the shoulder blade (photo **1**). Perform the upward movement with a slight pressure. First massage the left side seven times with the right hand, and then do the same massage for the right shoulder using the left hand for treatment.

**Circular massage with the thumb:** The left hand holds the shoulder, the right hand is on the left shoulder blade (photo **2**). Massage with your thumb with some pressure, which is just enough that your partner gets a sense of 'good pain' – that something good is happening which is dissolving tension. This may be experienced emotionally or physically.

Repeat the treatment format several times. Then change to the other side and treat it analogously.

**Circular massage with the palm of the hand:** Using the whole hand, now gently massage in circles over the point at the centre of the shoulder blade – the right shoulder blade 3 times clockwise and the left 3 times anti-clockwise.

Repeat the treatment several times.

**Circles over the shoulders:** Using both hands, now circle symmetrically several times over the shoulders (photo **3**).

**Treatment time:** 3–4 minutes.

## The shoulder–neck Marma – Amsa

Amsa means 'shoulder'. This tendon Marma is found in the area of the shoulders and neck.

**Application: Neck pain and tension, headache originating from the back of the neck, discomfort in the neck, anxiety.**

**Significance:** As a tendon Marma, Amsa gives resilience, will power and perseverance. But it can also be a place for anxiety and tension, worries and responsibilities: 'carrying a burden on the shoulders'. It is also an area where mentally undigested experiences and physically undigested food (Ama) accumulate.

**Control function:** The shoulder–neck Marma is related to the fifth or throat Chakra. It is the switching station for several energy channels that cross the Marma, and thus an important transit station for Pranic energy to the brain, and for the upward movement of Vata (Udana).

**Immediate effect:** Relaxation of neck, shoulders and arms. Relief from mental burdens.

**How to find Amsa:** Its centre is on the trapezius muscle, about a hand's breadth from the point at which the muscle is attached to the acromion bone. If you press here a little firmer with the middle finger, you will feel a sensitive area that radiates upwards to the neck and shoulder.

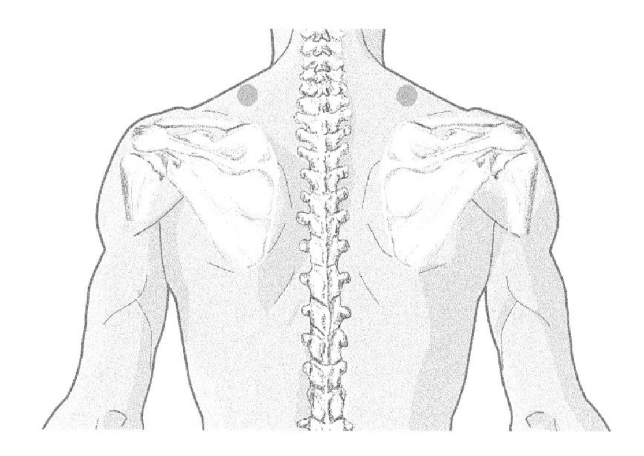

### OVERVIEW

**Marma type:** Snayu (tendon Marma)

**2 points:** 1 point on the left and 1 on the right shoulder

**Peripheral Marma:** on the palm, just below the gap between the index and the middle finger

**Effects:** controls the throat Chakra, gives perseverance, is a transit station for Prana moving in the Nadis to the head; deposit area for burdens and toxins (Ama)

**Oils:** muscle-relaxing oils include: MA 628 joint oil, sesame, almond, arnica, comfrey, Vata massage oil with Vata essential oil, jasmine, sandalwood

**Adhimarma:** Emotional Relief, Shanti Om, Sushumna

## Self-treatment

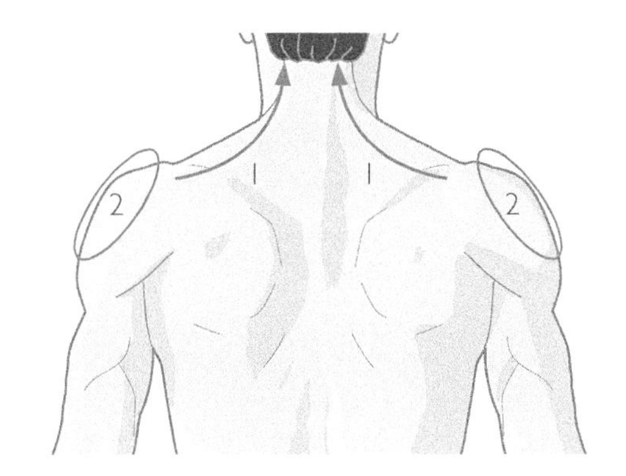


*Sequence and strokes for Amsa. In partner treatment the shoulders can also be treated (2).*

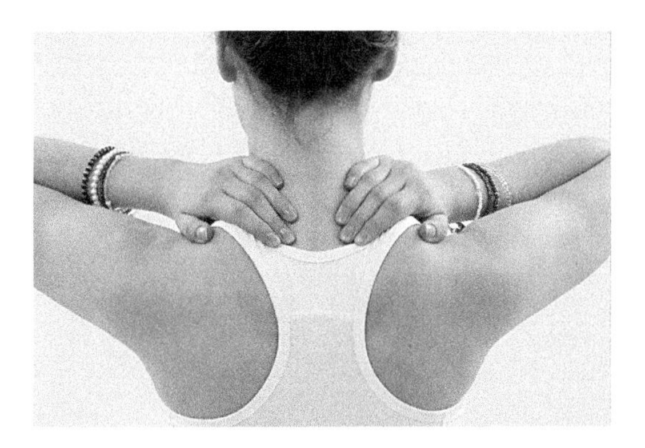

A firm massage of our own shoulders and neck with both hands simultaneously treats the Amsa Marma, which is located in the shoulders and neck. Put your hands on the area between the shoulders and neck and massage sensitively, with pleasure, from front to back (see illustration above). Relax periodically while massaging by allowing your hands to 'hang in' on the neck: the forearms will be parallel to the front of the chest, while the head is tilted slightly backwards and relaxed.

**Treatment time:** 3–4 minutes.

## Partner treatment

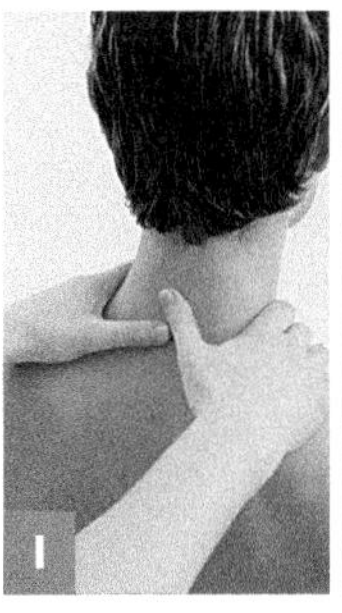


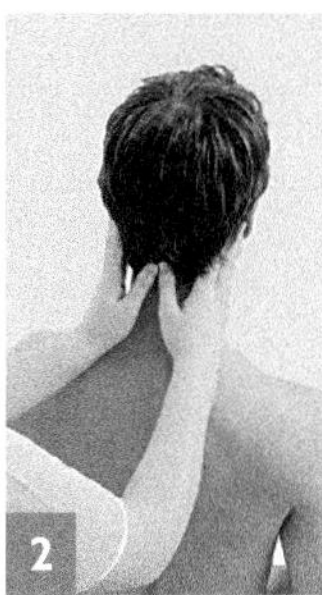


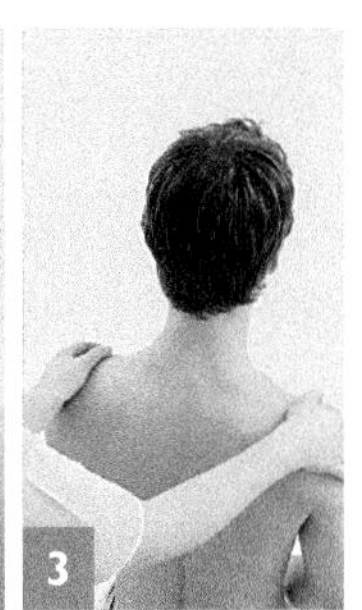


**Contact:** Stand to the left of your partner. Your left hand is a hand's breadth away from the throat and the right above the Amsa Marma (photo **1**).

**Up-and-down massage with the palm of the hand:** Your partner sits relaxed and comfortable and you stand behind them. Place your hands on the Marma and massage slowly in longitudinal strokes, calmly and gently, along the upper edge of the trapezius muscle, up to the neck and behind the ears (photo **2**). After seven strokes let your hand rest for about 10 seconds on the Marma. Repeat the process several times.

**Circles round the shoulders:** Using both hands, do a circling massage several times around the shoulders (photo **3**). Repeat the up-and-down massage described above.

**Hot towel compress:** This is a particularly effective way to end a treatment for neck tension: put half of the towel in hot (hand-hot!) water, wring it out and place it on the shoulder–neck region for half a minute. This can be repeated several times before towelling down with the dry half of the towel and letting your partner rest for a few minutes.

# Marmas of the Head and Neck

A great concentration of Marmas can be found on the head and neck. The head itself is considered to be one large Marma called Shiro Marma, and is the seat of perceptive and analytical consciousness. Sthapani, its centre, is the heart of the head, and Adhipati the supreme ruler. Along with Nila and Manya on the neck, these form the last three of the body's seven Mahamarmas.

Experience shows that a gentle treatment of the head and neck Marmas is particularly powerful and effective. Although most points in this area are fairly small, we can treat them easily with the thumb, index, middle or ring finger. However, extremely beneficial effects can also be achieved using the palm, for example in eye therapy, or using circular massage on the temple Marmas.

In Ayurveda the Marmas on the skullcap, Adhipati and Simanta, are treated with a variety of herbal oils depending on the constitutional type and the nature or cause of the health disorder.

The neck Marmas lie in soft tissue and therefore have to be treated very gently. Here we can use strokes with the hand over the whole area, which has the additional advantage that we don't have to locate the points accurately. In addition to the two energy pathways to the arms and legs and the six meridians which we discussed in the section on the back points related to the Chakras, six further Nadis are mentioned in Yoga literature. They all end at the head in Sthapani and supply the sense organs. Ida on the left and Pingala on the right rise up from the base of the spine and go to Sthapani, the third eye. From here they divide into four channels, two to the right and left eye (Pusha and Gandhari), and two to the right and left ear (Payasvini and Shankhini). This again illustrates the importance of Sthapani as the main Marma of the head.

Our ego is active in a special way in the Marmas of the face, neck, throat and head. These Marmas also mediate all our facial expressions, the whole display of emotions such as pleasure, pride, fear and sadness, or else a mask that hides our inner being. Their treatment can loosen deep-rooted blockages and bring out the beauty of our inner Being.

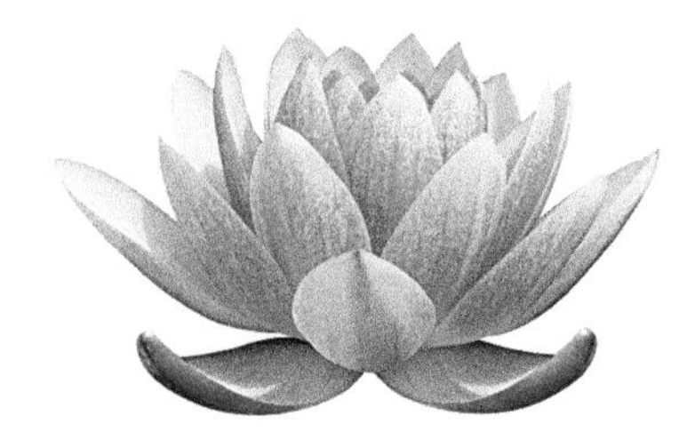

## THE SIX NADIS LEADING TO STHAPANI

**1 Pingala Nadi** – the fire element and Pitta Dosha dominate; it relates to the root Chakra and the sense of smell; it governs all Pitta activities including digestion and analytical and critical thinking; it supplies Prana to the right nostril and stimulates all the Marmas on the right side of the body.
**Main Marma:** Phana

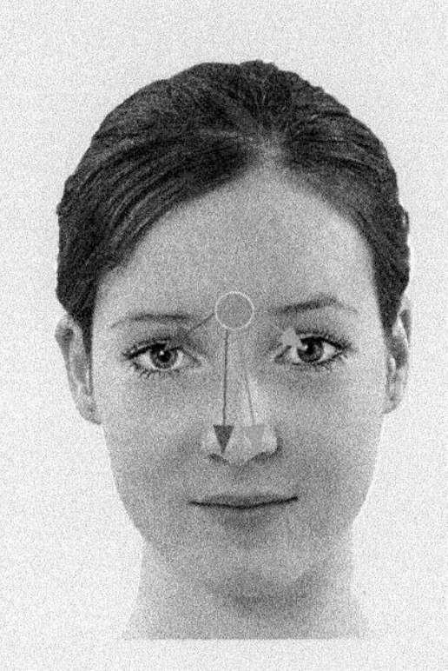

**2 Ida Nadi** – the water element and Kapha Dosha dominate; it relates to the root Chakra and the sense of smell; it governs all Kapha activities including the formation of body tissue, sleep and visionary thinking and speaking; it supplies Prana to the left nostril and stimulates all the Marmas on the left side of the body.
**Main Marma:** Phana

**3 Pusha Nadi** – supplies the right eye with Prana, the right eye being the seat of Atma in the waking state; it is related to Alochaka Pitta and the navel Chakra.
**Main Marma:** Apanga

**4 Gandhari Nadi** – supplies the left eye with Prana; enhances the experience of dreaming, creative vision and imagination; it is related to Alochaka Pitta and the navel Chakra.
**Main Marma:** Apanga

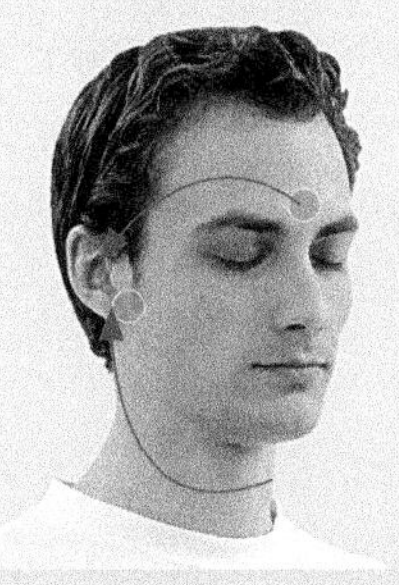

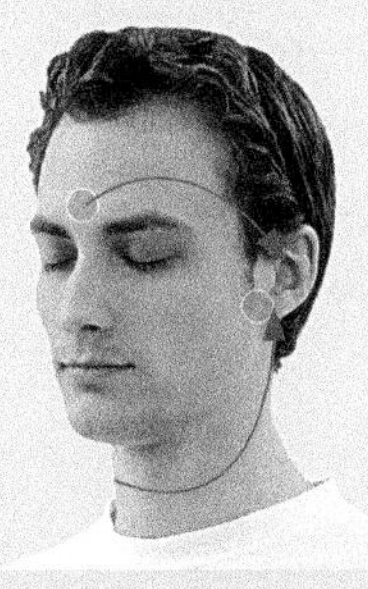

**5 Payasvini Nadi** – provides the right ear with Prana; conveys the inner perception of the sounds of the Veda; is connected to the throat Chakra which rules over hearing.
**Main Marma:** Vidhura

**6 Shankhini Nadi** – supplies the left ear with Prana; benefits devotion to higher, divine influences; is connected to the throat Chakra which rules over hearing.
**Main Marma:** Vidhura

## The neck Marmas – Nila, Manya and Sira Matrika

Nila means 'blue', and the name is derived from the blue translucent neck veins. The throat Chakra which is controlled by Nila is also described as having a blue aura. Manya means glory (which is bestowed on someone who is allowed to give a speech) but also 'jaw', which describes the location. Sira Matrika means 'mother of the blood vessels' and is an inner Marma that governs the blood vessels of the neck; it consists of four areas on each side of the neck along the carotid arteries.

**Application: Nila: thyroid disease, speech disturbance, hoarseness, swallowing problems, sorrow or anger that cannot be expressed or isn't allowed to 'shout out'. Manya: heavy tongue, excess flow of saliva or dry mouth, indigestion in stomach, colon and small intestine. Sira Matrika: autonomic dysfunction in the neck and circulatory disorders of the head.**

**Significance:** Nila is the Marma of language and free expression. It watches over everything that needs to be expressed in speech and action, from inside to outside. This Marma is disturbed when we have to swallow grief, when anger sits in the throat, or with the constricted feeling in the throat that we have when weeping is suppressed. In contrast, Manya has control over the tongue as the taste organ and also the glands that moisten it. Sira Matrika guards over the blood supply to the thyroid gland and the head.

**Control function:** Nila controls the throat Chakra, the thyroid gland, blood circulation to the brain and speech. It ignites metabolism, stimulates circulation and regulates blood flow to the skin (Brajaka). The meridians of the stomach, small intestine and colon which are controlled by this Marma, as well as the salivary glands, all run through Manya. Manya controls the water element and has predominantly Kapha features.

**Immediate effect:** Relaxation of the neck, a liberating feeling in the throat, clear voice, liberation of mucus in the throat.

**How to locate the neck Marmas:** Nila and Manya occupy large areas to the left and right of the larynx. Both Nilas are slightly above the thyroid to the right and left, and have a similar shape. Manya sits a little higher and to the side, under the mandibular angle. The eight Sira Matrikas lie between the two other neck Marmas along the carotid arteries, which you can gently feel with your fingers.

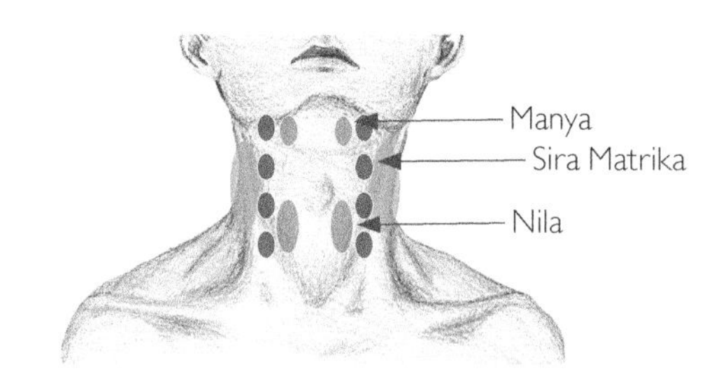


### OVERVIEW

**Marma type:** Sira (vessel Marma)

**12 Marma areas:** 6 on each side of the neck

**Peripheral Marma:** Kshipra

**Effects:** controls the fifth Chakra, speech and respiration (Udana), the salivary glands and sense of taste (Bodhaka), the heart and circulatory system (Vyana Vata), circulation (Brajaka Pitta), metabolism (Agni)

**Oils:** the following are soothing: Vata massage oil, Vata aroma oil; for heat, overactive thyroid and other Pitta disorders: Pitta massage oil and Pitta aroma oil are appropriate

**Adhimarma:** Nila/Manya, Udana

## Self-treatment

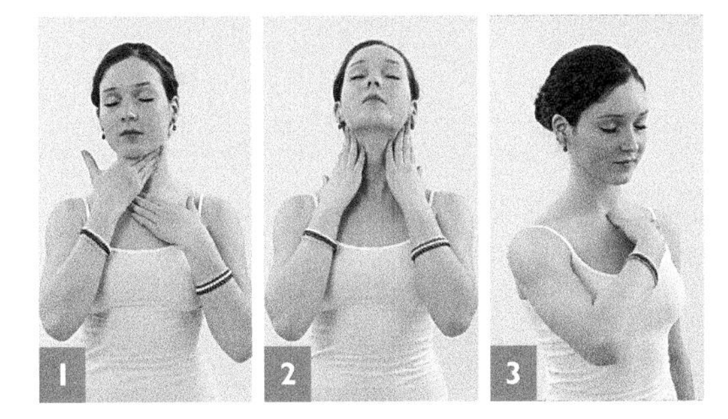


**Gentle smoothing massage:** In Ayurvedic oil massage, the neck is traditionally massaged in an upward direction, towards the head, using gentle, smoothing movements. In this way we not only reach both the neck Marmas, but also Sira Matrika, which is located at the side of the thyroid gland (see illustration). You can do this sitting up comfortably or lying down. Stroke alternately with both hands from the pit of the neck to the jaw, 10 to 15 times (photo 1).

**Up-and-down strokes on the side of the neck:** With the fingertips of both hands stroke the lateral neck up and down along the sternocleidomastoid muscle from the larynx to behind the ears (photo 2). Take your time: these strokes should be done in a very calm, sensitive and tension-releasing manner. If you don't like the feeling on the neck, then treat only the pit of the throat.

**Up-and-down massage of the pit of the throat:** Put the right hand on the sternum under the pit of the throat. Using the thumb of the right hand, do very quiet and gentle massage strokes up and down in the pit of the throat (photo 3). Seven strokes up and down – repeat if you wish.

**Treatment time:** 2–4 minutes.

## Partner treatment

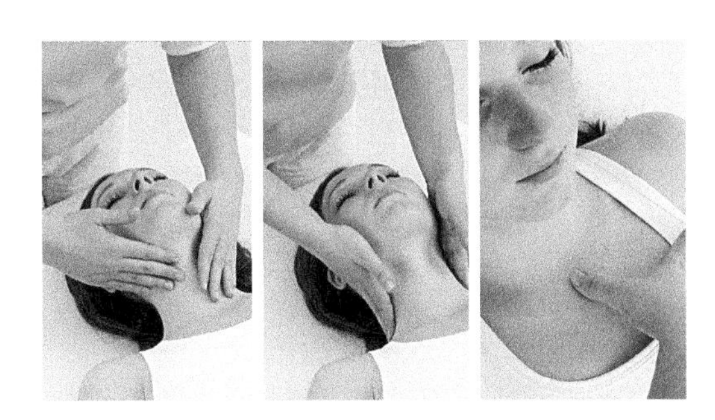

The treatment is similar to self-massage. Stand behind your partner, with hands and fingers positioned as outlined above. Especially here, if touching the neck is not tolerated, then treat only the pit of the throat. In this case, however, it is better if your partner is lying down.

**Contact:** Begin as always by making contact. If your partner is sitting, stand on their right with your left hand above the neck and the right over the throat. If your partner is lying down then the left hand is over the navel Marma (pages 74–75) and the right over the throat.

## The eye Marmas – Avarta and Apanga

Avarta literally means 'disaster', because the point is very sensitive. Apanga means 'on the outer corner of the eye'. Around each eye there are other Marmas that are also known in TCM as acupuncture points.

**Application: Eye strain, defective vision, headache resulting from strained eyes, blocked nose.**

**Significance:** The eye Marmas provide the visual system with Prana and control its energetic functions. Farsightedness is a quality of a free mind which can look into the future and can live and act with foresight. Long-sightedness (hyperopia) prevents us seeing the things that are immediate. Short-sightedness (myopia), in turn, has, as its potential background, the fear of being seen and criticized.

**Control function:** Avarta is a Sandhi (joint) Marma, although in a strict sense the point is not directly on a joint. However, in general, Marmas cover larger areas and the orbit is formed of several skull bones which allow subtle movements between each other. Avarta controls Vata, especially Prana Vata for vision, as well as Alochaka, the Subdosha for inner and outer vision. But even nasal breathing is affected. Apanga is a blood vessel Marma. It regulates blood flow to the eye and also vision. Its centre is the first point of the energy path of the gall bladder. In addition to Avarta and Apanga, there are other smaller points that strengthen the eyes as well as the paranasal sinuses and digestive organs.

**Immediate effect:** The treatment clarifies vision, relaxes and refreshes the eyes, calms the mind and relaxes the neck.

**How to find the eye Marmas:** Avarta is about thumb-sized. Its centre lies in the middle of the eyebrow. There you will feel a small, somewhat sensitive pit. Apanga can be found at the outer orbital rim, where the upper and lower edge of the orbit meet. Additional points lie on the opposite side of each of these Marmas, on the inner corner of the eye and in the middle of the lower orbital rim, where you may find a small hole for the nerve exit. The Bindu, the centre of the eye Marma, can be found by touching the eyelid very gently just over the pupil with the eyes closed.

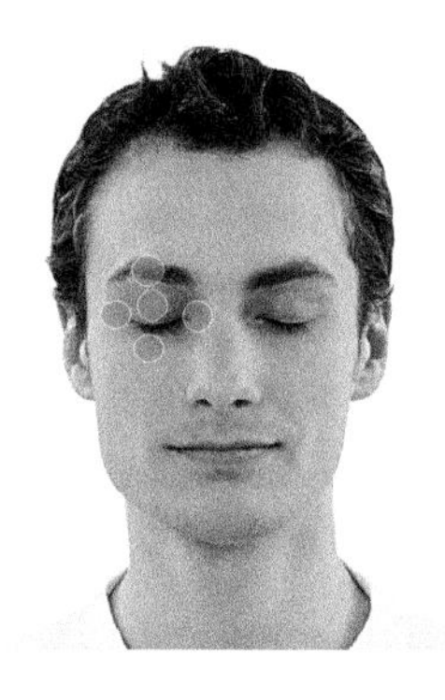

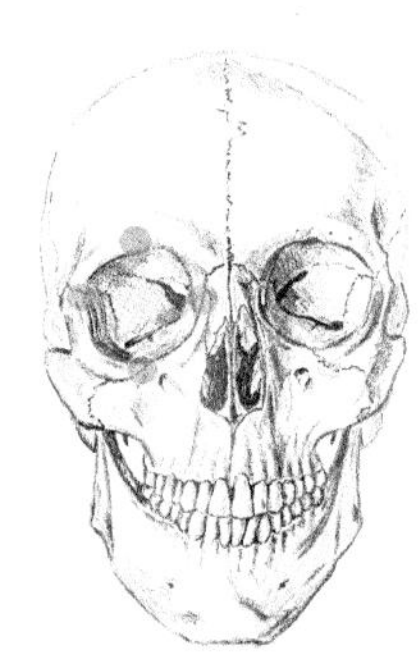

### OVERVIEW

**Avarta:** *Marma type:* Sandhi (joint Marma)

**Apanga:** *Marma type:* Sira (vessel Marma)

**4 points:** 1 Apanga and 1 Avarta point on each eye

**Peripheral Marma:** Kshipra between ring and little finger on both hands

**Effects:** Avarta controls Vata, Prana and Alochaka; Apanga controls Alochaka and Prana

**Oils:** ghee, triphala ghee, MA 550 Ghrita, sandalwood, rose, Pitta massage oil (cooling influence)

**Adhimarma:** Alochaka P, Alochaka V

## Self-treatment

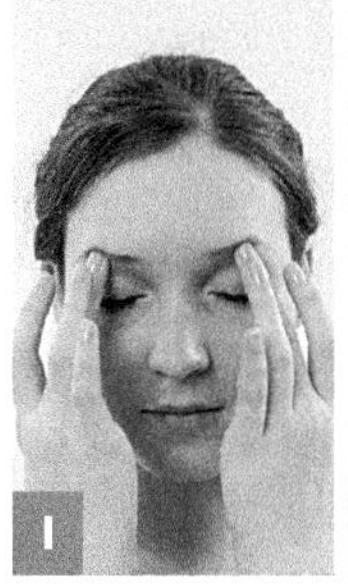


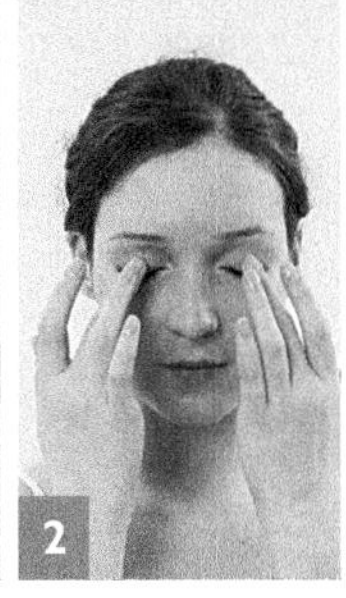


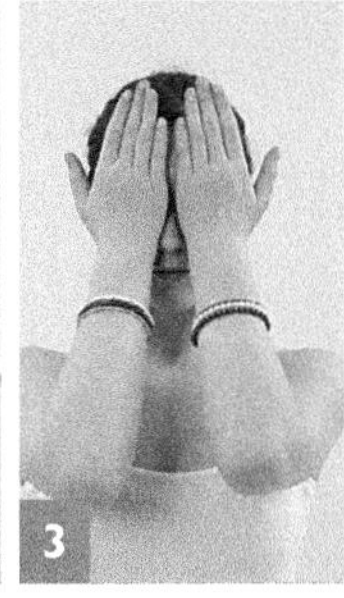


**Circling the eye:** Sit upright comfortably and keep the eyes closed throughout the treatment. Place the tip of your middle fingers at the corner of the eyes on the Apanga Marmas and massage very gently, both simultaneously and slowly on the left and right side around the inside edge of the eye socket (photo **1**). Stop at each point with a short, light pressure, and then continue. Massage three times to the right and three times to the left.

**Circular massage on individual Marmas:** Do three circles on each of the five eye Marmas (including the Bindu). Start at the inner eye points, proceed to the upper eye point, to the outer one and the lower one, and finally on the closed eyes, right over the pupils (photo **2**).

**Massage with the whole hand:** Now treat all eye points simultaneously with the flat hands. Rub your hands together vigorously to produce heat. Place them over the eyes so that the centre of the palm is on each pupil (photo **3**). The eyes are not totally closed. If the hands rest properly, then you will be looking into the darkness of your palms which lightly touch the eyelid. With calm and small circles, now massage around your eyes, from inside to outside in the case of short-sightedness; from outside to inside in the case of long-sightedness; and, if both vision disorders are present, do one cycle in each direction.

**Palming:** For 1–3 minutes allow your hands to rest over the closed eyes, with the middle of the palm on the eyes.

**Cotton pads with rose water:** Finally place cotton pads soaked in rose water (rose hydrolat) on the eyelids. Rest for 10 minutes.

## Partner treatment

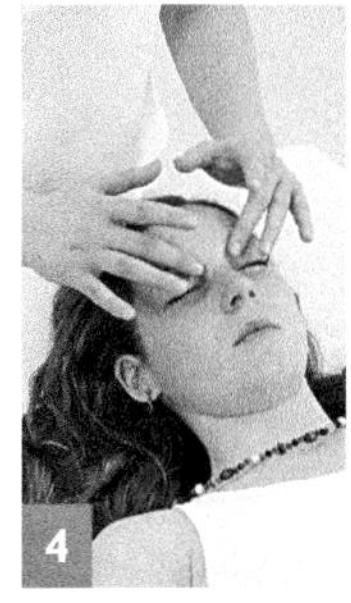


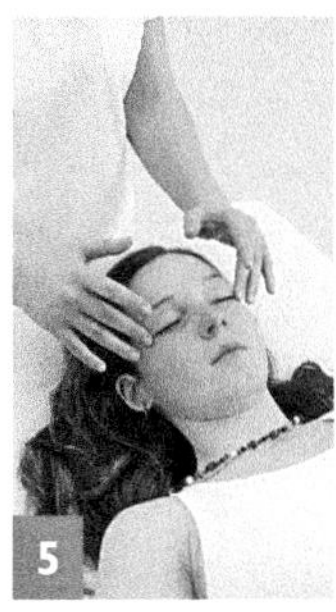


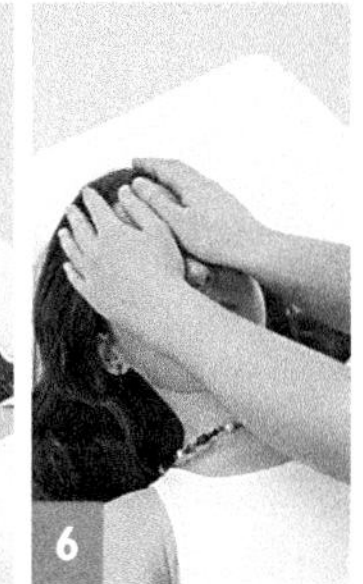


Partner treatment is performed in the same way as self-treatment. Your partner lies relaxed on their back and you stand behind them (photos **4**, **5**).

**Contact:** Right hand over the navel Marma (solar plexus, strengthening Agni), with the left above the eyes.

**Completion of treatment:** Place your palm on the eye sockets of your partner, and let them rest for one or two minutes, giving warmth (photo **6**). Finally, place cotton pads soaked with rose water onto the eyelids and let your partner rest with the pads for 10 minutes.

## The ear Marma – Vidhura

The Sanskrit word Vidhura literally means 'pain' and this point is very sensitive. But Vidhura is also a famous sage, the embodiment of virtue. In the famous Indian epic, the *Bhagavad Gita*, Vidhura gives wise counsel to a blind ruler, but the advice falls on deaf ears and this results in war.

**Application: Deafness, tinnitus, neck pain, ear pain (also where this is caused by a blockage of the first cervical vertebra), anxiety.**

**Significance:** The word 'hearing' is ambiguous: it means the process of acoustic perception of our external world through the ear; on the other hand, if we do not want to listen and are tired of hearing something or a person, then this reflects the psychological side of our hearing. This Marma is a very alert radar antenna directed both inward and outward.

**Control function:** Two large and important Nadis (Payasvini and Shankhini) end at the ear Marma. The side extension of the first cervical vertebra lies just below this point. This Marma controls the fine adjustment of the head by the neck muscles for optimal perception and controls Vata.

**Immediate effect:** During the treatment you can get the feeling that the ear is opening up and hearing is becoming clearer. Sometimes you can feel an energy beam to the third eye and then from the forehead over the top of the head (along the bladder meridian).

**How to find Vidhura:** The Marma is behind the earlobe, in front of the temporal bone. When opening the mouth, the finger falls into the pit behind the ear. Next to it is the approach of the sternocleidomastoid muscle on the temporal bone. In front of the ear, above the jaw joint, is another effective ear Marma point ('Sevikuthi' front ear Marma, Triple Heater 21 in TCM). You can find it when you open your mouth and the fingers fall into the pit of the jaw.

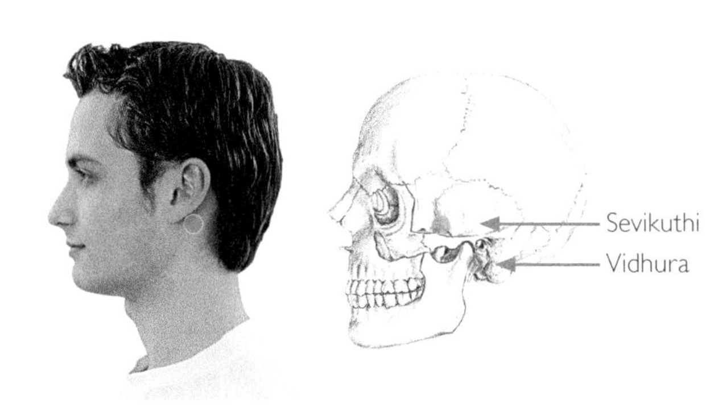


### OVERVIEW

**Marma type:** Snayu (tendon Marma)

**2 points:** 1 point each on the left and right ear

**Peripheral Marma:** Kshipra, especially the point between the index and the middle finger and between the fourth and little toe (pages 56–57)

**Effects:** clears hearing, awakens Prana in head and ears

**Oils:** Vata massage oil mixed with Vata aroma oil, basil (calming); clarifying oils, for example in sinusitis and deafness: Kapha massage oil with Kapha essential oils, pine, anise, eucalyptus

**Adhimarma:** Adhiprana, Sushumna, Basti, Emotional Release

## Self-treatment

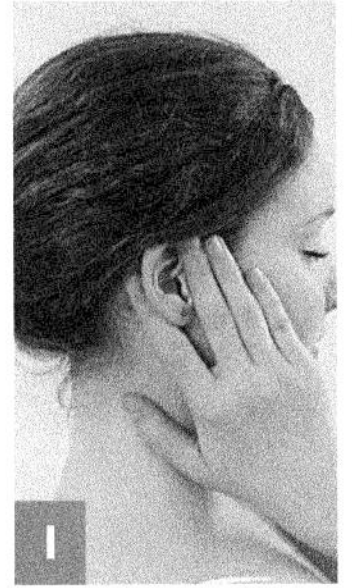

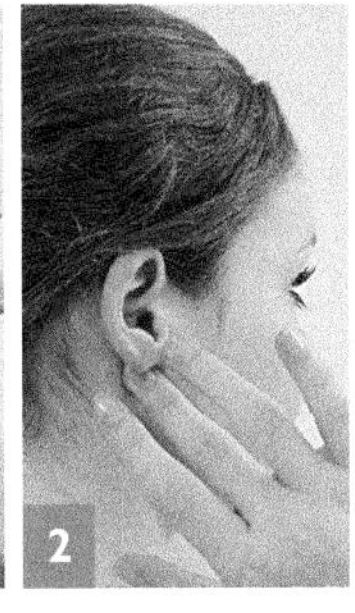

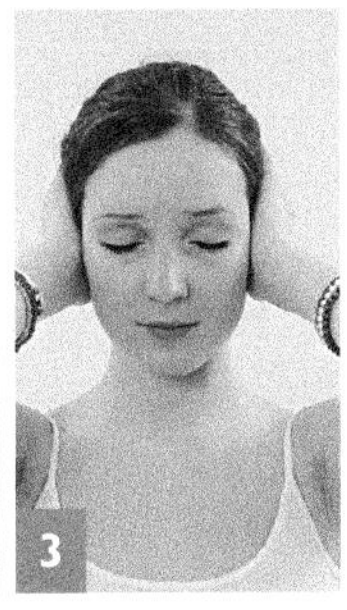


**Up-and-down strokes in front of and behind the ear:** Remove any ear jewellery. Sit comfortably upright and treat both ears simultaneously. With the middle finger directly in front and the index finger behind the ear, massage gently three times up and down (photo 1); you can repeat this three times. At the end of the downward movement of each cycle, let your middle finger rest for about 10 seconds on the vital point in front of the ear and the index finger on Vidhura Marma.

**Circular massage on the Marma:** Massage both the Vidhura points gently with the tips of the two middle fingers (photo 2). Repeat several times.

**Circles over the ears with the palms of the hands:** Place your hands flat on the ears, and make very gentle and quiet movements in a clockwise direction (relating to the right ear) (photo 3). In between, let your hands rest on the ear for about 10 seconds and enjoy the warmth and relaxation.

**Completion of treatment:** Place your palm on the ears and enjoy the gentle warmth and energy that flows from the hands for one or two minutes.

**Treatment time:** 3–5 minutes.

## Partner treatment

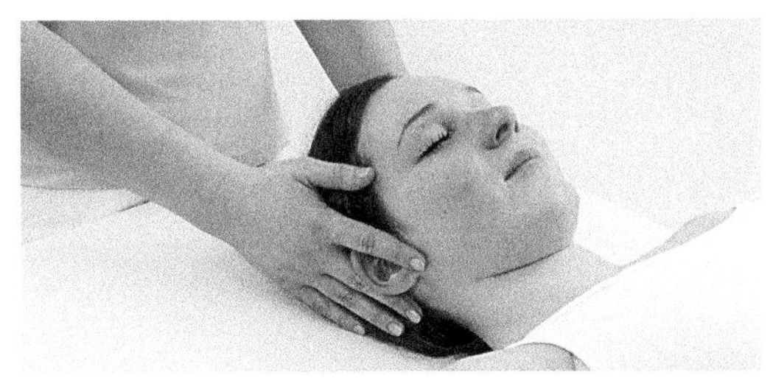

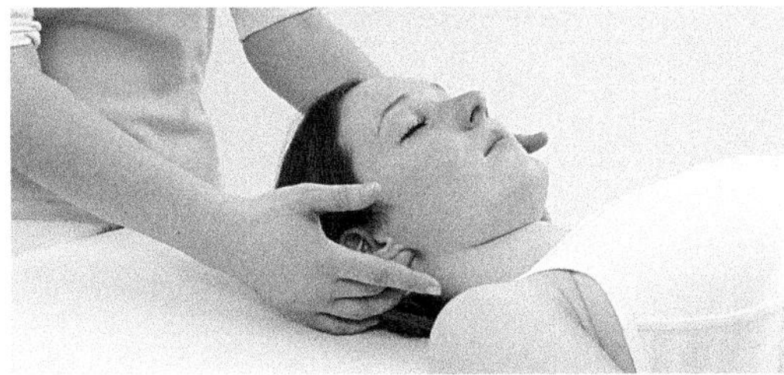

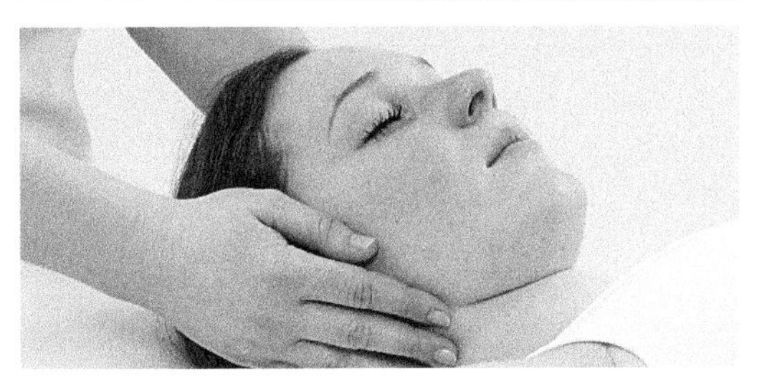

Your partner (wearing no earrings) relaxes. Proceed in the same way as self-treatment. Below are the only differences.

**Contact:** Stand behind your partner with your left and right hand a hand's breadth away from the ears (for two to three breaths).

**Up-and-down strokes:** The index finger is in front and the middle finger is behind the ear (top picture). At the end of the last downward movement let your index finger rest over the jaw joint in front of the ear (vital point for the ear) with the middle finger behind the ear (for about 10 seconds).

## The neck Marma – Krikatika

The Sanskrit word literally means 'neck joint'. It is the connection between the first cervical vertebra and the atlanto-occipital articulation.

**Application: Neck tension, neck pain, stiff neck, blockage of the first and second cervical vertebrae, pain in the back of the head, anxiety, shoulder pain.**

**Significance:** Krikatika Marma is the guarding awareness on the gate to the head. It protects, gives warning, controls and opens the doors of perception for all the senses. Fear is located here in the neck, as well as pride and self-confident straightforwardness. Because of its key role and its location, this Marma is involved in almost all the functions of the organs of the head and spine as well as in posture.

**Control function:** When we treat Krikatika we affect many vital points left and right of the spine that belong to the bladder meridian. The paired bladder meridian starts at the root of the nose, passes over the head down the whole spine, continues down the back of the legs and ends on the outside of the little toe. If there is a blockage of Krikatika Marma (for example, in the joint of the first cervical vertebra), the functions of the whole meridian on the same side as the blockage can be delicately disturbed.

**Immediate effect:** Relaxation of the neck muscles, a fresh feeling in the head, clearer sight, calmer mind.

**How to find Krikatika:** The two Marma areas are found at the junction of the cervical spine on the occiput, left and right, just below the occipital protuberance. There is a very important central Marma that connects and integrates both these points and it is located between them where the back of the neck meets the skull. In Siddha medicine it is called Pitari (neck) Marma. TCM calls it Fengfu (palace of the winds). It is opposite Sthapani, the third eye, and is its corresponding point.

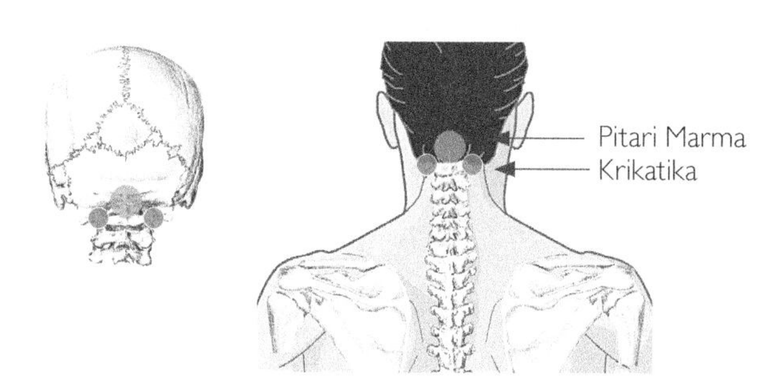


### OVERVIEW

**Marma type:** Sandhi (joint Marma)

**2 points:** 1 point on the left and right of the neck

**Corresponding Marma:** Nila/Manya

**Effects:** controls the flow of energy to the head (Prana), the unconscious reflexes and function of the central nervous system and nutrients to the brain (Tarpaka); controls body position and monitors the upward movement of Vata (Udana)

**Oil:** Vata oil, almond oil, Dhanvantari oil, MA 628 joint oil (for neck pain), joint soothe oil.

**Adhimarma:** Sushumna, Udana

## Self-treatment

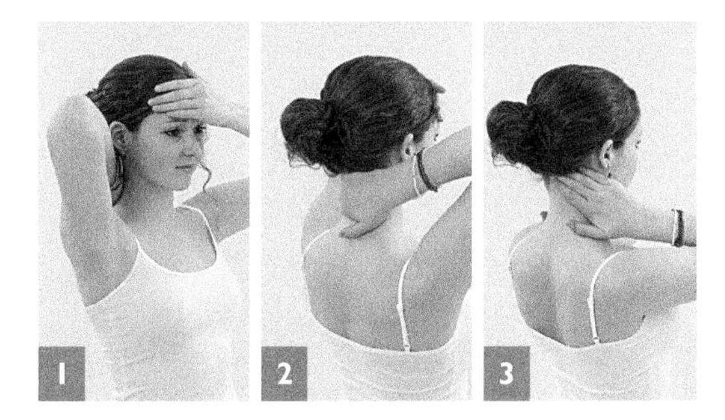

**Circular massage with the palm of the hand:** The treatment is simple but effective, even if you only massage with a dry hand without oil. For a painful or stiff neck or neck headache, the best oil is MA 628. In this treatment we also include the shoulder–neck Marma Amsa (pages 88–89) and small Marmas along the spine. Place your left hand on the forehead with the centre of the palm on the Marma of the third eye. It is the counterpoint to the two Krikatika Marmas. Gently and calmly massage in a clockwise direction with the right hand over the occipital protuberances (photo 1).

**Up-and-down strokes along the neck with one hand:** Massage with the right hand on the neck, rubbing up and down, from the upper neck to the back of the head (photo 2). Do this about 20 times or as many times as is comfortable.

**Vigorous rubbing:** After sitting for long periods and strenuous mental work, quickly rubbing tense neck muscles distributes the accumulated energy and brings immediate relief.

**Up-and-down strokes along the sides of the neck with both hands:** Massage with the flat hands on the sides of the cervical spine from the shoulder to behind the ears 7 to 10 times up and down (photo 3). This massage can also be done with more pressure, as long as it feels good.

**Completion of treatment:** If there is neck pain, put a warm compress on the neck and repeat 2 to 3 times.

**Treatment time:** 3–5 minutes.

## Partner treatment

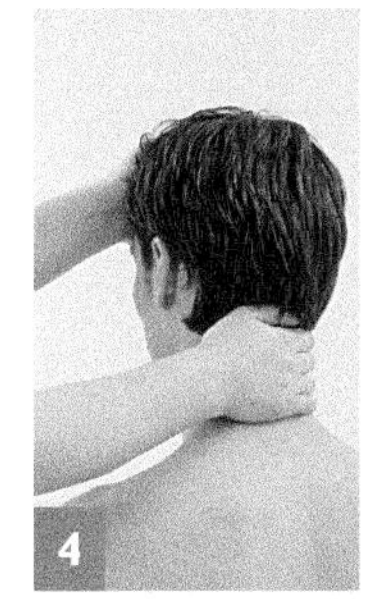

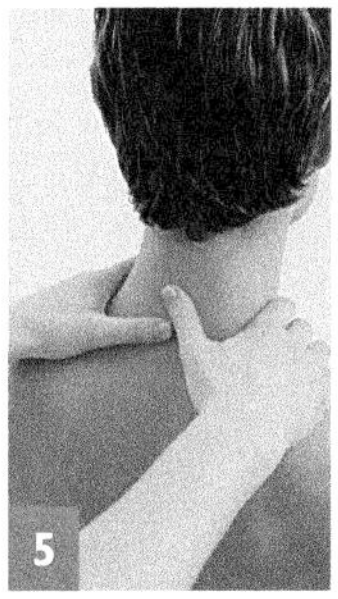

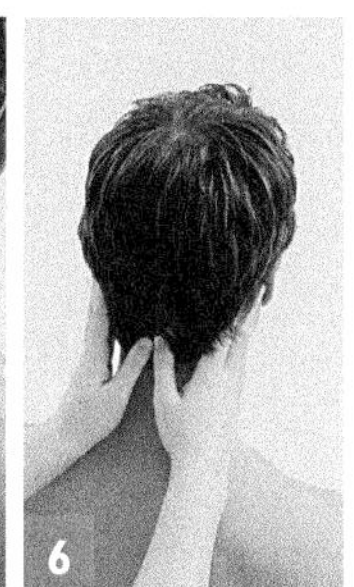

This is similar to self-treatment but with the following differences.

**Contact:** Stand to the left of your partner. Your left hand rests a few inches above the Marma of the third eye, with your right hand over the neck Marma (two or three breaths) (photo 4).

**Up-and-down strokes along the sides of the neck with both hands:** Massage 7 to 10 times up and down from the shoulder to behind the ears with the hands flat on the sides of the cervical spine. The hands are not oblique, but directed upwards. The fingers lead the movement up and follow it down (photos 5, 6).

**Completion of treatment:** For neck pain put a warm compress on the neck – repeat this 2 to 3 times.

## The temple Marmas – Shankha and Utkshepa

Shankha means 'conch shell', like the shape of the temporal bone. This bone Marma is very sensitive. Utkshepa means 'that which drives upwards'. This tendon Marma lies above the temple Marma, on the temple muscle.

**Application: Headache in the temples, dizziness, nausea, mental overexertion, teeth grinding, sleep disorder through anger or strain, nasal congestion, rhinitis, strained eyes, gall bladder ailments.**

**Significance:** If we exert ourselves mentally and 'bother our head' about something, the temple Marma comes into play. Shankha Marma is the monitoring awareness of the most fragile and sensitive part of the skull. The temple is a region of Pitta, of fire energy. If we get angry, blood pounds in the arteries in the temples. Utkshepa opens the flow of energy upward towards the temple Marma. It gives relief. Shankha is an area where strenuous thinking takes place, while Utkshepa harbours a more uplifting and lighter awareness.

**Control function:** Several meridians cross on both Marmas with links to bile, stomach, eyes, ears and nose. Utkshepa is the gate for Prana to flow up to the crown Marma.

**Immediate effect:** Calms the mind, relaxes the facial muscles (especially the jaw muscles), allows mental burdens to drop away, opens the nose, relaxes and refreshes the eyes (especially when using ghee).

**How to find Shankha and Utkshepa:** Shankha lies on the temporal bone in the middle between the corner of the eye and the upper attachment of the ear (see photo below). If you place three fingers here, you can feel the pulse of the temporal artery. Utkshepa is three fingers above. The area is often slightly painful to touch. If you open and close the mouth, you can feel the tension of the temple muscle.

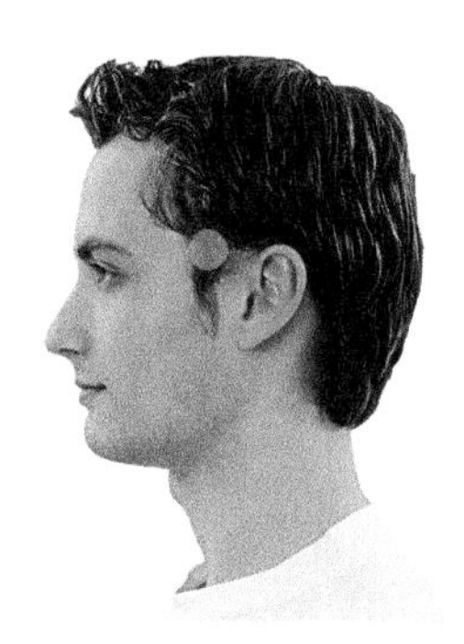

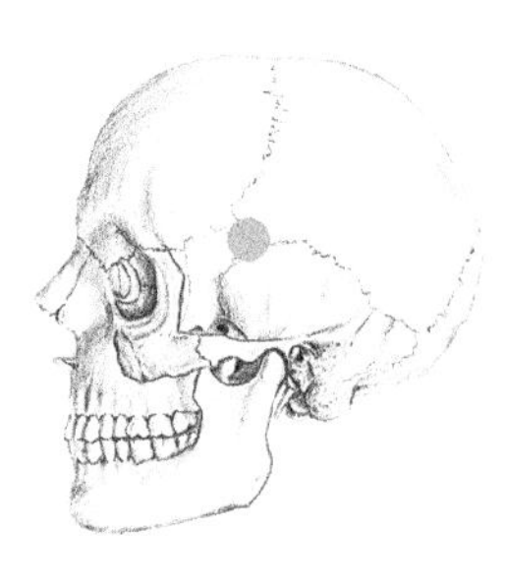

### OVERVIEW

**Shankha:** *Marma type:* Asthi (bone Marma)

**Utkshepa:** *Marma type:* Snayu (tendon Marma)

**4 points:** 2 points on each temple

**Central Marma:** Sthapani, Adhipati

**Effects:** Shankha monitors emotional Pitta, liver and bile, Apana Vata in the colon and Prana in the brain. The centre for the sense of touch, which lies in the cerebral cortex, lies next to this Marma, which supports its functioning. Utkshepa brings Prana upward and has an effect on the salivary glands (Bodhaka) and the sense of smell

**Oil:** Vata oil, almond oil, lavender, rose, mint oil, Pitta oil, ghee (Pitta-cooling)

**Adhimarma:** Adhipati, Sthapani, Hridaya, Emotional Relief (Sadhaka)

## Self-treatment

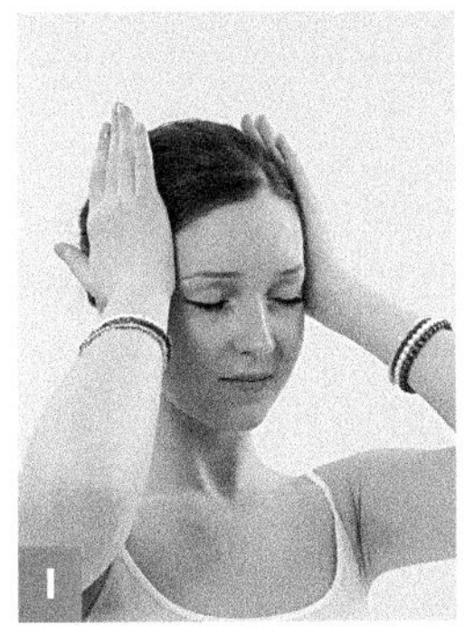

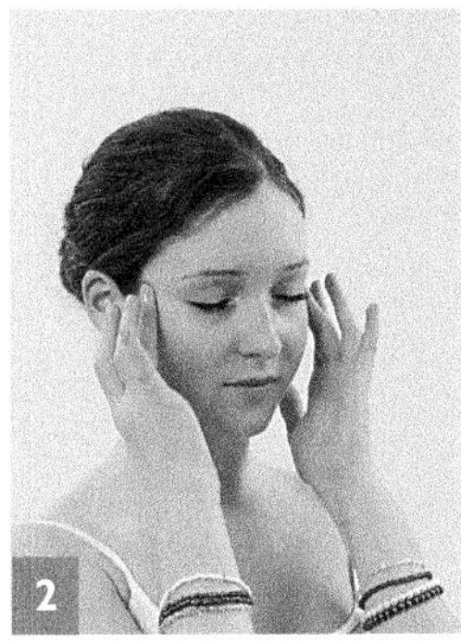

Do circles over the temples: with or without oil the treatment is very relaxing and liberating. What follows is the treatment of Shankha, but Utkshepa is treated similarly. Sit upright or lie comfortably on your back. Put your hands on your temples, with the palms just above the points, and very quietly and gently massage in circular movements (photo **1**). You can move the skin a little over the temporal bone, which in many cases is even more relaxing.

Repeat the 1–3–5–7 treatment format several times.

**Massage with three fingers:** Very gently and softly massage the two points with the index, middle and ring fingers in a circular motion (photo **2**).

Repeat the treatment format several times.

**Completion of treatment:** Place your hands for one or two minutes on each temple and give the Marma peace and energy.

**Treatment time:** 3–5 minutes.

## Partner treatment

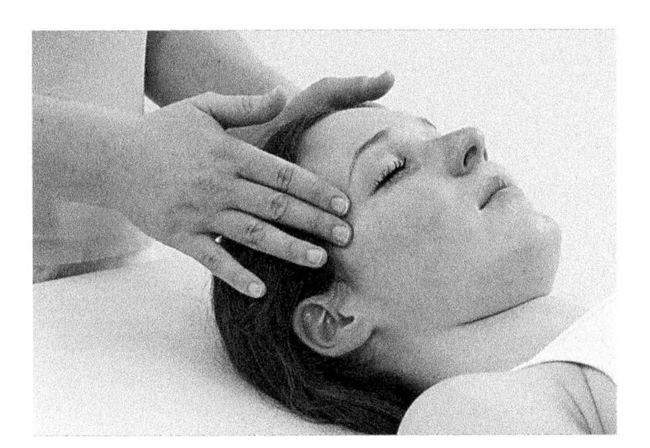

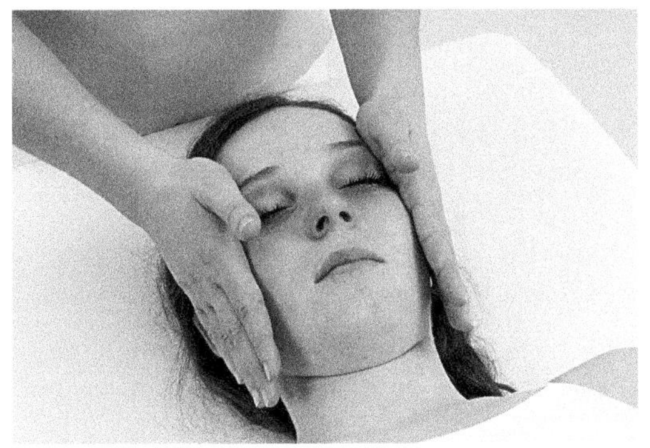

The treatment is similar to self-treatment.

**Contact:** Your partner lies comfortably on their back. Stand or sit behind them. Lay your hands in a soothing way either on their temples or a little distance away.

## The palate Marma – Shringataka

Shringataka describes the shape of an antler or a place where four streets intersect. It is the meeting point of four pranic energy channels for perception, namely the tongue, nose, eyes and ears. The Marma includes four areas on the soft palate.

**Application: Nervous weakness, taste disorders, disorders of the salivary glands, disturbance of vision, hearing and smell.**

**Significance:** The palate is, after vision, smell, touch and hearing, the last important supervisory control unit before food, liquids, breathing air and other materials enter through the mouth into the body. Because of this the Marma has a very important function: it monitors the quality of what we bring into the body, and coordinates it with the other senses. To have a sense of taste – good or bad, even in a psychological sense – lies within the consciousness of this Marma.

**Control function:** From the Ayurvedic perspective we absorb Prana from food via the palate and this Marma, which then forwards it to the senses and organs. Even the word *Prana* itself is articulated so that in the '*n*' the tongue is placed against the palate (palatal consonant). This touches the source of Prana and enlivens it. The soft palate is also an important point for concentration and meditation; it controls all the senses and supports the flow of Soma or nectar from and to the crown Chakra. It is described as the place of the moon, which absorbs the nurturing Soma or Kapha. In contrast, the navel Marma is the seat of the sun and of Agni, the digestive fire and vitality.

**Immediate effect:** Strengthening this Marma revives and regenerates; it reorders thinking and recharges all the 'batteries' of the body, hence all the Marmas.

**How to find Shringataka:** Put your tongue against the palate – this is the Marma. Two corresponding points lie outside the mouth, left and right below the zygomatic arch, where the eye socket nerve emerges from a small pit (see illustration).

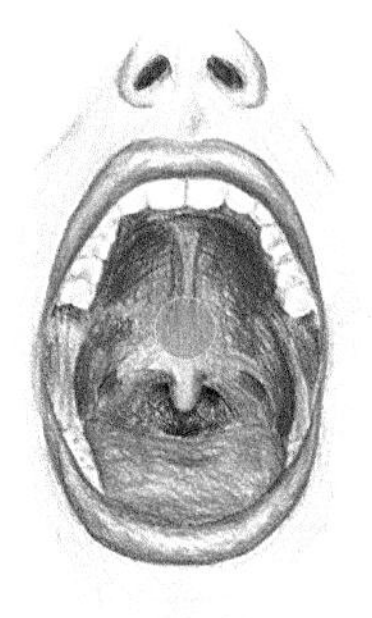

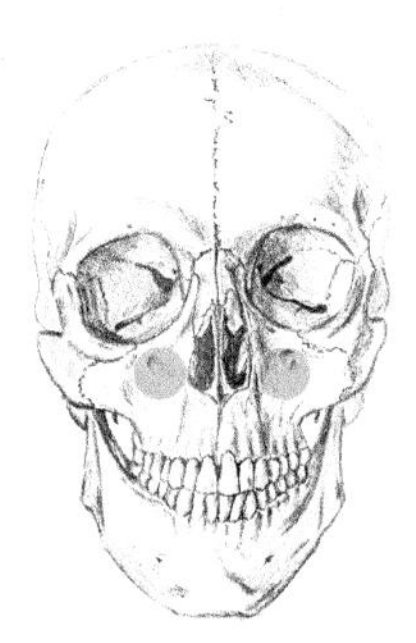

### OVERVIEW

**Marma type:** Sira (vessel Marma)

**4 areas:** on the soft palate

**Peripheral Marma:** the tips of all five fingers

**Effects:** nourishes all the senses and organs with Prana which is absorbed from food; strengthens the sense of taste and the salivary glands (Bhodaka) and the nervous system (Tarpaka); absorbs Ojas and supplies the organism with this nourishing fluid

**Oils:** Vata oil and Brahmi oil to strengthen the nerves

**Adhimarma:** Udana, Adhiprana, Emotional Relief

## Self-treatment

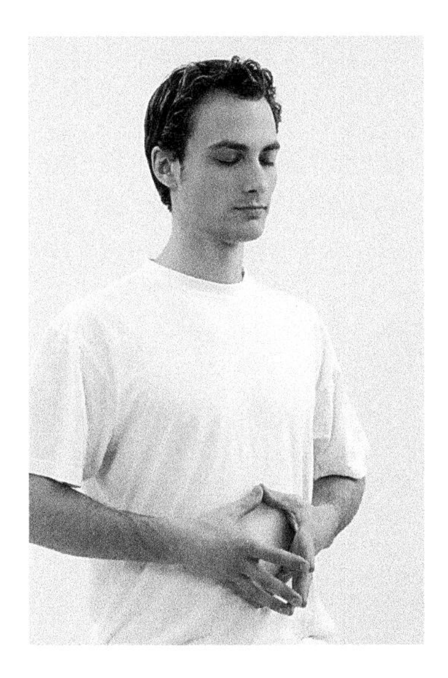

**Treatment with the tongue; strengthening with Mudra:** Sit upright comfortably, close your eyes and put the tongue on the palate. Fold the hands to Hakini Mudra in front of the navel (see page 75 and the photo above). Breathe naturally and quietly and have your attention on the tongue and palate.

**Treatment time:** 3–5 minutes.

## Partner treatment

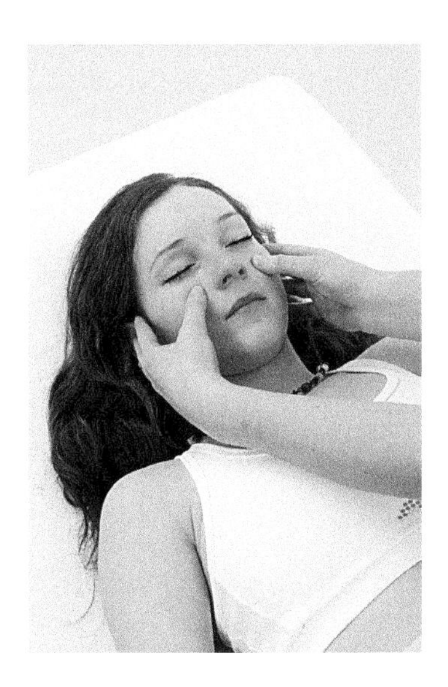

To treat the palate directly is experienced as unpleasant. While your partner is internally enlivening and strengthening the Marma as in self-treatment, you can harmonize and strengthen the corresponding point on the cheeks with soft, calm, circular movements using your thumbs (see photo above).

Repeat the treatment format several times.

**Treatment time:** 2–5 minutes.

## The third eye – Sthapani

Sthapani means 'that which is steady and stable, giving strength and direction'. The third eye is the centre and 'heart' of the head.

**Application: Nervousness, insomnia, hormonal disorders, headache in the forehead, overstrained eyes, visual impairment, worry, grief, anxiety, excessive concentration, narrow-mindedness, nervous heart complaints and also for strengthening self-confidence.**

**Significance:** In Sthapani the seeing consciousness for inner knowledge, vision and analysis is located. It is the centre of the senses and the mind. It also has the feeling insight of the heart (Sadhaka). When we ponder, worry, become annoyed or cannot let go mentally, the forehead becomes wrinkled and the eyebrows squint together to express the emotional burden of Sthapani. Its treatment gives inner peace and opens the heart for love and compassion, but also strengthens clear thinking, courage, confidence, inner happiness and emotional intelligence and takes away the anxiety that leads to *short-sightedness* and therefore bad choices and decisions.

**Control function:** The third eye controls the sixth Chakra (Ajna) and the six Nadis of the head (page 90 and the following) that emanate from it, and provides the eyes, ears and nose with Pranic energy. In addition it acts on the pituitary gland. Since the pituitary is superior to all other hormonal glands, this Marma is generally hormone regulating and therefore has a very wide-reaching influence on the functions of the body as well as on the state of mind. Thus winter depression is a consequence of lack of light on this Marma, for sunlight stimulates it. Sthapani rules inner light, the light of consciousness, and governs the fire (Agni) of the mind and the senses.

**Immediate effect:** Strengthening of this Marma calms thinking, relaxes the eyes, refreshes the mind and gives immediate peace.

**How to find Sthapani:** It is located slightly above and between the eyebrows. Another point with similar characteristics, the centre of the sixth Chakra, lies at the centre of the forehead ('Netri Marma', the Marma of the middle of the forehead). Sthapani is connected with it. Both are included in the treatment.

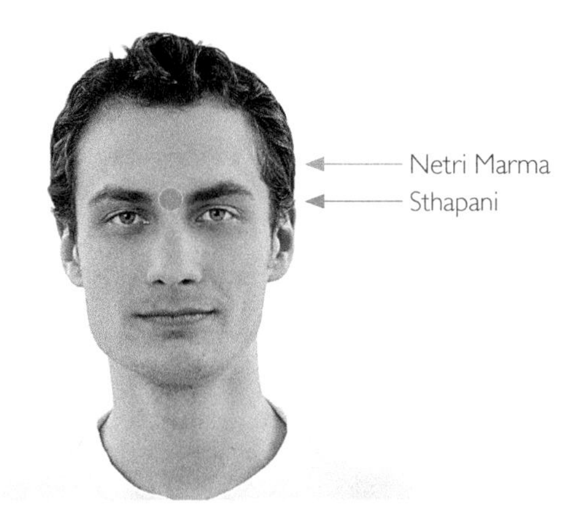


### OVERVIEW

**Marma type:** Sira (vessel Marma)

**1 point:** between the eyebrows

**Peripheral Marma:** Marma of the tip of the thumb which manifests itself in Gyan Mudra (page 114).

**Effects:** controls the sixth Chakra (Ajna), Prana, mind, senses and pituitary, the six Nadis to the third eye, Sadhaka Pitta and Tarpaka Kapha

**Oils:** sandalwood, lotus, basil, rose (calming, cooling and opening); saffron (hormone-regulating); mint, eucalyptus (refreshing and strengthening)

**Adhimarma:** Sthapani

## Self-treatment

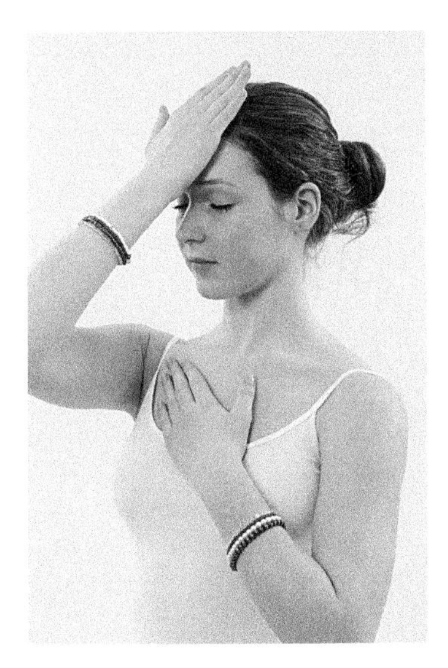

**Circular massage with the palm of the hand:** Sit comfortably upright, close the eyes and put your right hand with the centre of the palm on the Marma and the left one on the heart. Perform a gentle, calm, circular massage; from your point of view this is anti-clockwise (from the front seen as clockwise).

Repeat several times. At the end of the last cycle leave your hand on the point for a few breaths and enjoy the silence. Then relax for a few minutes.

**Treatment time:** 3–5 minutes.

## Partner treatment

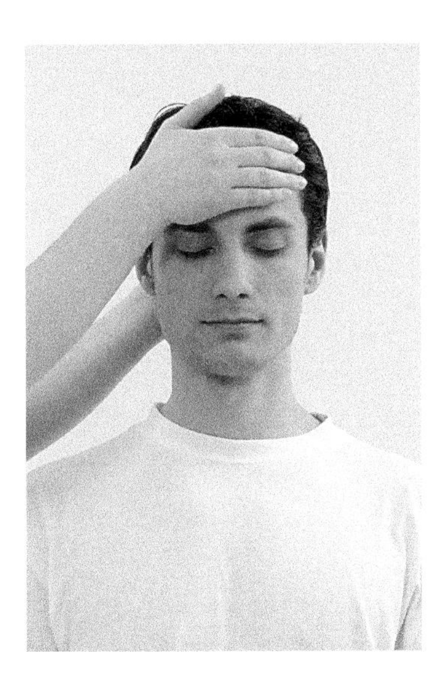

**Contact:** Stand to the right of your partner with your left hand on the back of their head and the right one a few inches in front of the forehead. You may either touch the forehead and the back of the head or maintain a distance according to the well-being of your partner. Sometimes, if the forehead has become hot as a result of stress and over-thinking, it feels good to first apply to the forehead a cool, damp cloth soaked with rose water and to start the treatment after the forehead has cooled down and become calmer. Then treat as described in self-treatment. Gently support the junction of head and neck (Krikatika Marma) with your left hand.

**Treatment time:** 2–3 minutes.

## The crown Marma – Simanta

Simanta means 'the peak' – the skull roof and its seams. It is a joint Marma on the cranial sutures.

**Application: Nervousness, insomnia, anxiety, fatigue, headache, neck tension, circulatory insufficiency.**

**Significance:** The crown Marma covers the brain like a protective helmet and monitors its various areas and parts. The skull bones are slightly moveable at their seams, and these joints allow an adaptation to consciousness processes and physical changes that act on the head.

**Control function:** The crown Marma controls the seventh Chakra (Sahasrara), the nervous system, plasma, blood and circulatory system and thinking, similar to Adhipati, which is in its centre and is superior to it.

**Immediate effect:** Vigorous massage of the Marma refreshes and invigorates, eliminates fatigue, clears the mind and stimulates circulation. Gentle massage is relaxing, removes mental stress and enlivens feelings of happiness.

**How to find Simanta:** The Marma consists of five areas and has an unusual shape and extent. It sits on the connections or seams of the skull: the long centre seam, the front left and right side (coronal suture) and the rear left and right side (lambda suture).

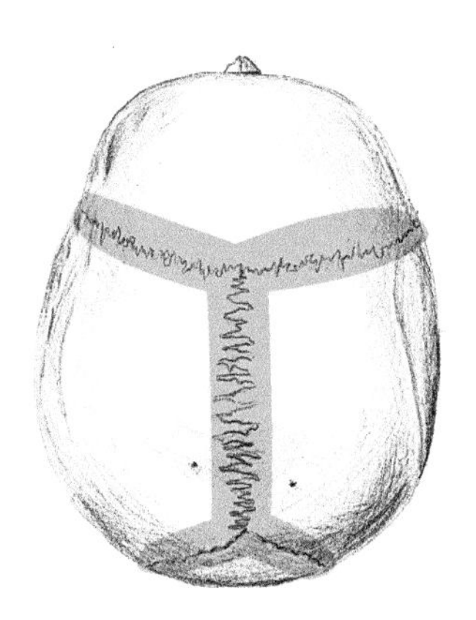

### OVERVIEW

**Marma type:** Sandhi (joint Marma)

**1 point:** comprises 5 areas

**Peripheral Marma:** manifests in the fingertips when they form a Mudra.

**Effects:** controls the seventh Chakra (Sahasrara), nervous system (Tarpaka), Prana and circulation (Vyana)

**Oils:** for a calming and tonic effect use Vata massage oil with Vata aroma oil, Brahmi, lotus, jasmine, valerian

**Adhimarma:** Adhipati

Self-treatment

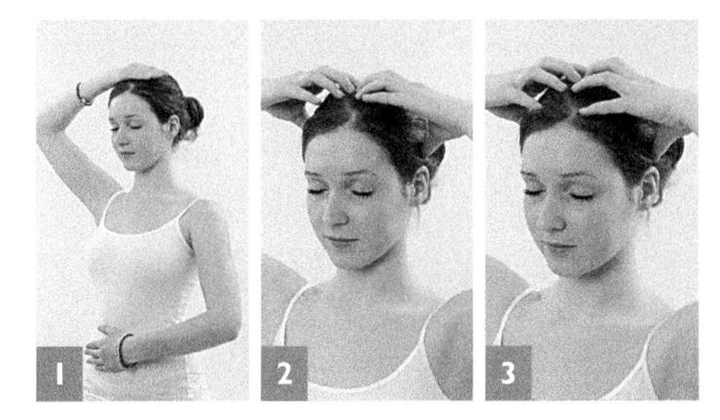


**Circular massage with one hand:** There are various ways to treat this Marma. In India it is normal to massage the head strongly because it is considered an organ of Kapha. You could try this. But we would again recommend using a gentle method, which has an effect on a deeper level of the physiology and on the level of consciousness. Begin in the same way as for treatment of Adhipati (pages 108–109) with a gentle, circular massage on the top of the head (photo **1**). Repeat several times.

**Massage along the centre seam:** Continue along the longitudinal seam in the centre by massaging slowly and gently with the fingers of both hands along the centre line from back to front and back (photo **2**). Repeat several times.

**Circular massage on the front and rear seam:** Finish with a massage of the front cranial area, making circles as if you are washing your hair, with the thumbs resting on the temples. Massage the back of the head in the same way. Here it is best if the thumb rests on the occipital protuberances (photo **3**). Always go with your feeling and well-being; it must simply feel good. If you use oil, then leave the oil after the massage for between a few minutes and half an hour before taking a shower. After treatment with oil avoid going outdoors if it is cold.

**Treatment time:** 3–5 minutes.

Partner treatment

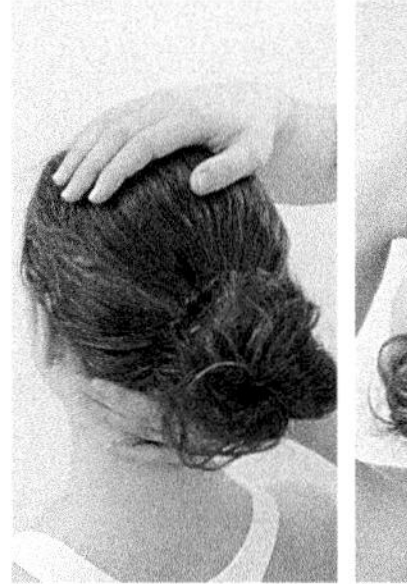
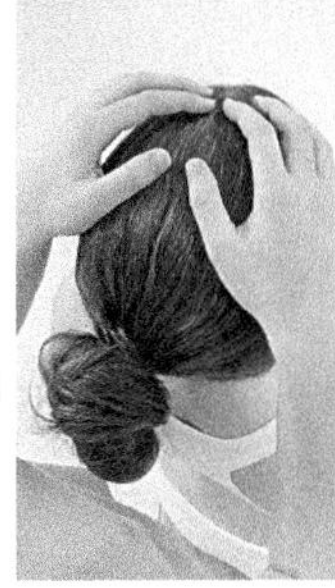
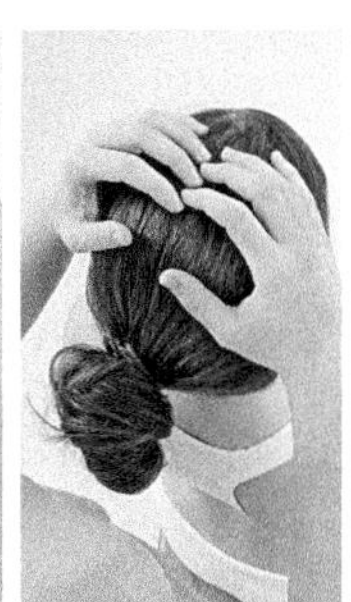

Massage in the same way as for self-massage. The hands and fingers will be set differently, of course. Choose what feels to be the most comfortable technique for you.

**Contact:** Stand behind your partner. Both hands rest a few inches above the head protecting it from above and the sides.

**Treatment time:** 2–3 minutes.

## The crown Marma – Adhipati

Adhipati is known as the 'supreme ruler'. Due to its position at the top, like the president of a country, this Marma ensures that the government rules according to its constitution.

**Application:** Nervousness, insomnia, anxiety, fatigue, confused thinking, headache.

**Significance:** Through the crown Marma we experience intuition. When this Marma functions harmoniously, we have an overview of the full spectrum of our daily tasks and goals. From the lofty seat of the watchful consciousness of Adhipati it is easy to maintain the overview. If the coherence in the consciousness of this Marma becomes disrupted, then we become disoriented and lose ourselves in the diversity of the world.

**Control function:** The crown Marma controls the seventh Chakra (Sahasrara), the pineal gland, the nervous system as a whole, lubrication of the brain, the energy of thinking, feeling (Sadhaka) and the primary elements of life for health, happiness and strength (Ojas, Agni and Prana).

**Immediate effect:** Strengthening this Marma calms and clears thinking, refreshes the mind and awakens feelings of peace and happiness.

**How to find Adhipati:** It is on the top of the head in the middle of the skull roof at the juncture of the sutures (see picture below).

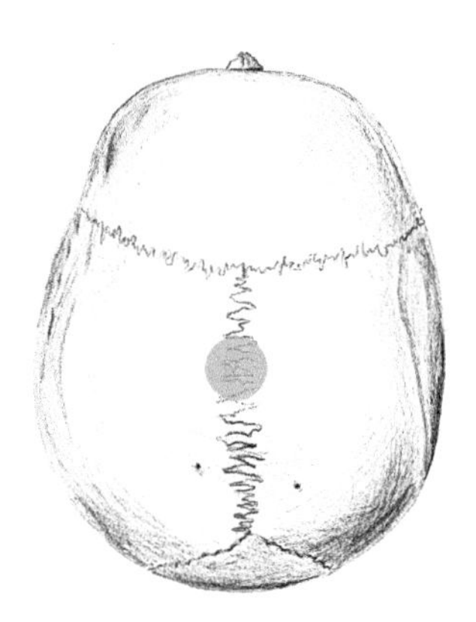

### OVERVIEW

**Marma type:** Sandhi (joint Marma)

**1 point:** at the top of the head, in the area of the frontal fontanelle

**Peripheral Marma:** fingertips of thumbs, index, middle and ring finger in the gesture of the Adhipati Mudra (see page 113)

**Effects**: controls the seventh Chakra (Sahasrara), pineal gland, nervous system (Tarpaka), Prana, Agni and Ojas

**Oils:** Vata oil, Vata aroma oil, sesame oil, Dhanvantari oil, Brahmi oil

**Adhimarma:** Adhipati

Self-treatment

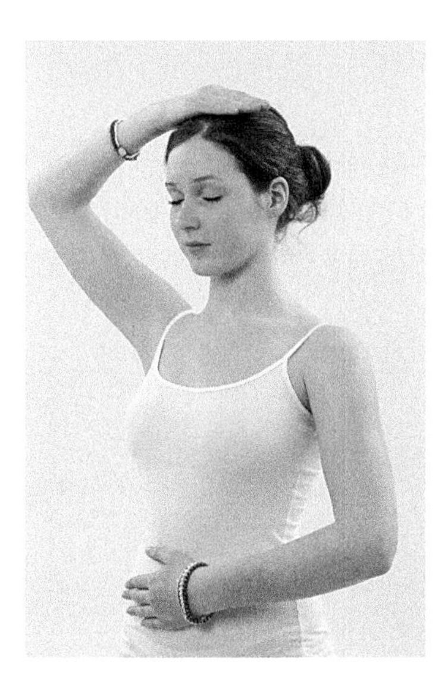

**Circular massage with the palm of the hand:** Sit comfortably upright, close the eyes, and place your right hand with the centre of the palm on the Marma. The left hand is placed over the heart or the navel. Do a gentle, calm circular massage in a clockwise direction. Repeat several times.

At the end of the last cycle allow your hand to rest on the Marma for a few breaths and enjoy the silence. Relax for a few minutes.

**Treatment time:** 3–5 minutes.

Partner treatment

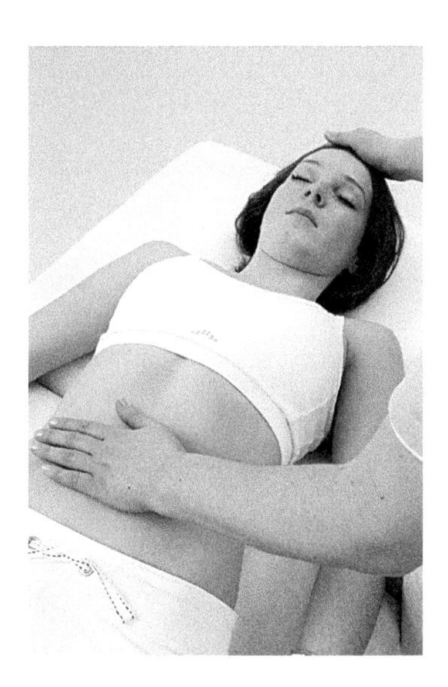

This is similar to self-treatment. Your partner sits upright or lies comfortably on their back.

**Contact:** If your partner is sitting, then you stand to their right with your left hand above their upper back at the height of the shoulder blades above the Brihati Marma (pages 84–85). Your right hand rests over the crown Marma. Keep a few inches' distance, as being too close can be perceived as unpleasant pressure. During the treatment your left hand will touch and assist the Brihati Marma.

If your partner is lying down then stand to their left with your left hand over their navel and the right above the crown Marma. Treat with your right hand, as shown in the illustration above.

# Mudras and Marmas

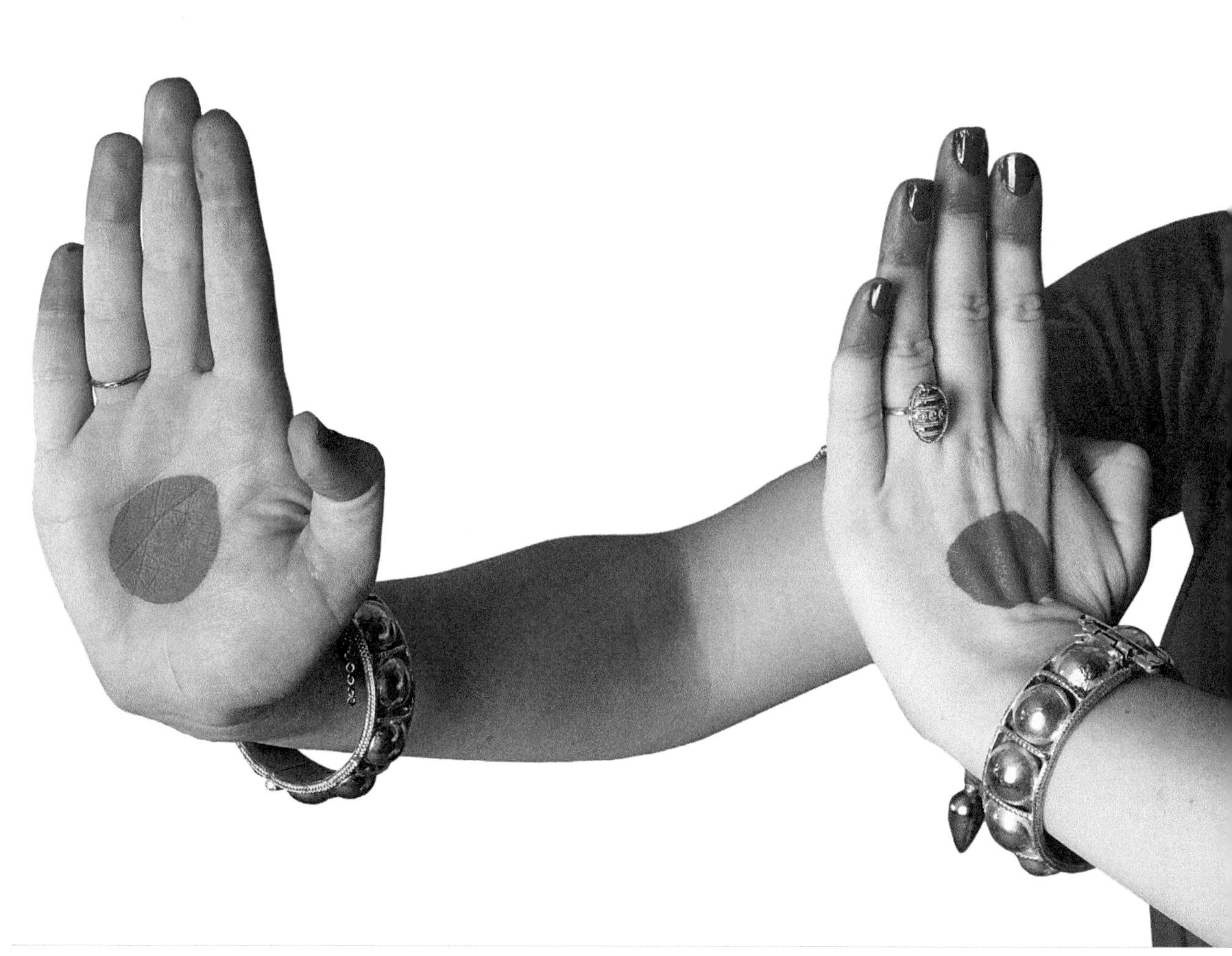

# Conscious Gestures Lead Inwards

*Mudra* means 'sign' or 'seal'. A Mudra is a posture or gesture through which we spontaneously express our feelings or state of consciousness in everyday life. If we feel reverence or esteem, we intuitively fold our hands as if in prayer. Similarly, if we want to pray, we fold our hands for devotion and to collect ourselves by moving our attention inward, to ourselves.

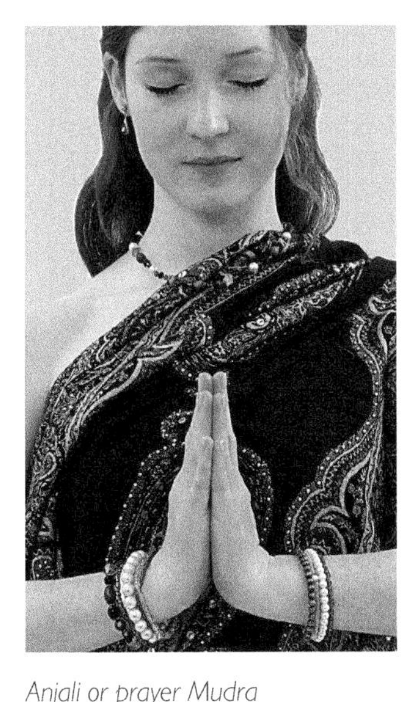

*Anjali or prayer Mudra*

Mudras and Marmas are closely connected. Awareness expresses itself as a Mudra, and a Mudra – a gesture, a posture that we adopt consciously – in turn creates this state of consciousness. Through a Mudra we can correct disorders in the Marmas, raise their status and strengthen their functioning. If we perform a finger, hand or body posture in a certain way, specific Marmas get ordered, protected, enlivened or calmed. We therefore use Mudras to support and complement a Marma treatment.

## Attention improves the effect

To be able to feel the subtle energetic changes in the body consciously, one needs attention, peace and a contemplative attitude. Sit upright, but comfortably. Close your eyes for one moment and breathe deeply. Then perform the appropriate Mudra and without expectation feel what happens in your body or in your consciousness. To get a feeling for the specificity of the energy of a finger gesture you can gently rub your fingers for a moment, as you would if you were testing a piece of silk for quality.

## Each Mudra has its grace

Each Mudra expresses a particular state of being and has its own beauty. Feel the specific quality that each Mudra generates in the mind and the subtle changes that take place in your body. Initially it may require a certain degree of patience to feel the flow of energy which a Mudra generates in the body. The first sign that a Mudra is being performed correctly is often the feeling that the nose opens up and breathing becomes freer. Prana begins to flow. But even if you do not feel anything, the Mudra still has its effect and brings about the desired changes.

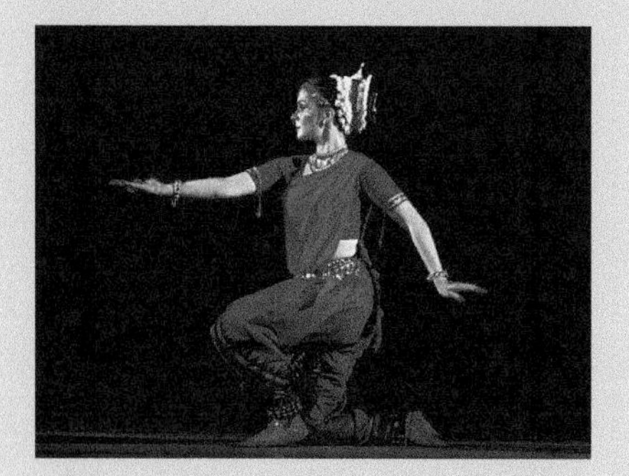

## MUDRAS IN INDIAN TRADITIONAL DANCE

Classical Indian dance dates back to the period of Vedic culture and is an aspect of Gandharva Veda, the knowledge of the healing effect of the sounds and melodies of nature. Gandharva Veda is expressed in singing, with musical instruments or in dance. Mudras play a highly significant role in dance. The feeling and content of the dance – which always tells a story of the great Indian spiritual tradition – finds its expression in the gestures, the specific Mudras of Indian dance.

## Understanding the effects of the Mudras

We can understand the effect of various Mudras better if we appreciate their influence on the Marmas, the energy channels, the five elements, the Doshas and Subdoshas, as well as the reflex zones of the hands and feet. In the example of the meditation Mudra (Gyan Mudra, photo **1**; page 114), this can be easily illustrated: the tip of the thumb and index finger touch each other, forming a closed circle which incorporates the Kshipra Marma (pages 44–45). The two energy channels of colon and lungs meet in Kshipra, and Pranic energy gathers here as if in a basin, strengthening this Marma. We have already described this confluence of energy pathways, the Sangam, on page 18. Similar effects occur with the other hand Marmas like Talahridaya (pages 46–47), which is incorporated into the circulation of the flow of energy through the opposite positioning of thumb and middle finger (photo **2**), or thumb and ring finger.

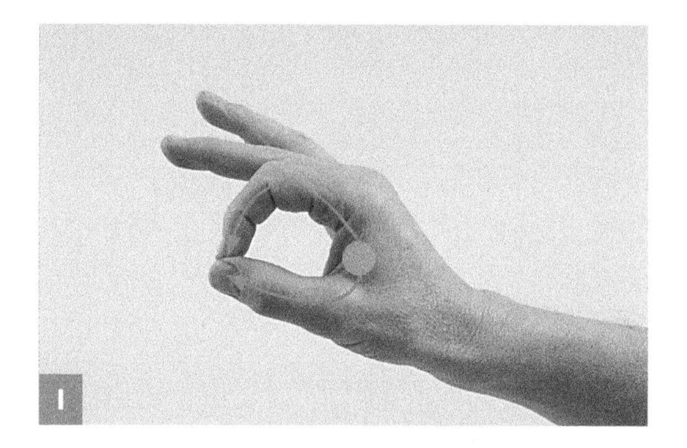

*Confluence (Sangam) of the Nadis of colon and lungs in Kshipra*

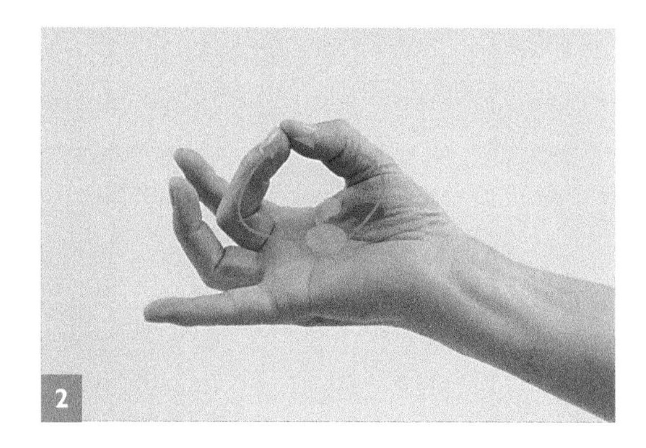

*Confluence of the Nadis of circulation and lungs in Talahridaya*

## Mudras and Doshas

We can also understand the effect of a Mudra from the relation of the fingers to the five elements, the *Mahabhutas*, and the three Doshas (illustration below right). The three Doshas Vata, Pitta and Kapha, derived from the combining of the five elements, manifest respectively on the index, middle and ring fingers. How we form a Mudra with the 'Dosha fingers' determines its effect on the three bioregulators and their sub-functions, the Subdoshas. The Prana Subdosha, for example, is located principally in the fingertips and especially in the thumb. Anyone who has strong Prana has great healing power in his or her hands. Prana can be felt as the vibrant energy of the aura that we can perceive when someone's hand comes closer to our body and penetrates our aura.

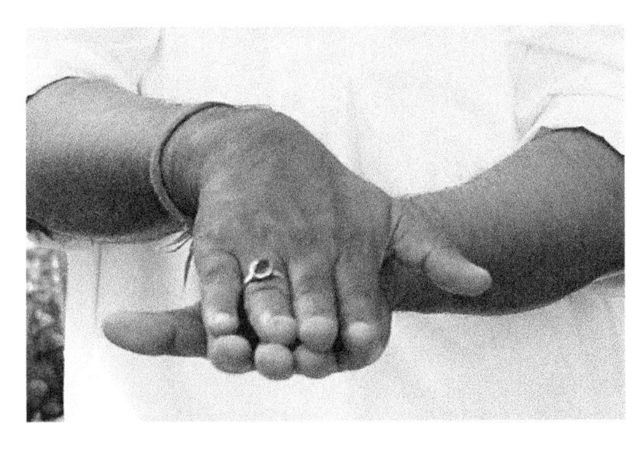

*The 'Fish' Mudra*

## Mudras manifest Marmas

Since the hand reflects the whole body in miniature form, we also find here a correspondence to all the other Marmas in the body, comparable to the representation of physical organs on the reflexology zones of the hand. Thus we find a correlation between Adhipati (pages 108–109) and the tip of the thumb. The Marma manifests itself when we put the thumb (which represents totality) together with the index, middle and ring fingers (the representatives of the three Doshas) to form a Mudra, while stretching out the little finger.

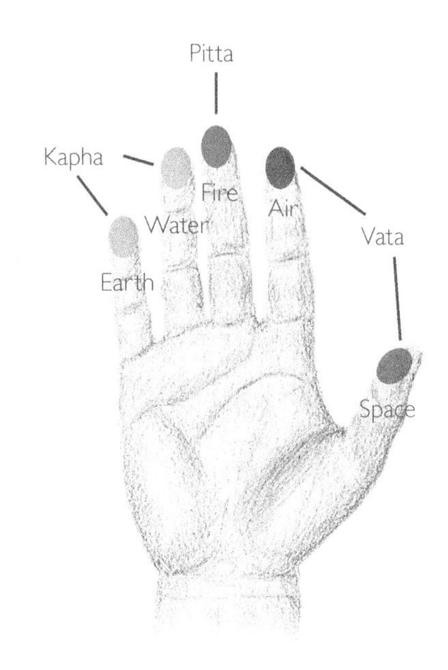


*The five elements and the three Doshas on the hand*

## Finger Mudras

### Meditation or Gyan Mudra

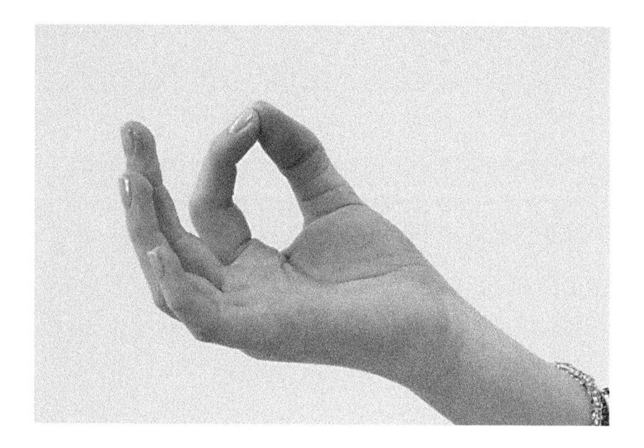

**With each hand:** Place the tips of the forefinger and thumb together and hold your hands open with the palms facing upwards.

**Effect:** Supports contemplation and meditation, gives precision in thought and action, helping to find the correct word; strengthens digestive fire (Agni) and gives contentment to the heart (Sadhaka); and helps in respiratory diseases (Udana). Reduces fatigue, especially when the thumb and forefinger are pressed together during inhalation and then relaxed during exhalation.

The ethereal elements of space (Akasha) in the thumb and air (Vayu) in the index finger dominate this Mudra, which is why it raises consciousness and promotes lightness in thinking.

**Marmas that are involved and strengthened:** Adhipati (tip of the thumb), Kshipra (Sangam of the energy path of index finger and thumb), Kurcha and Kurchashira (contraction of the ball of the thumb).

**Practice time:** 5–10 minutes twice daily.

### Sun or Akash Mudra

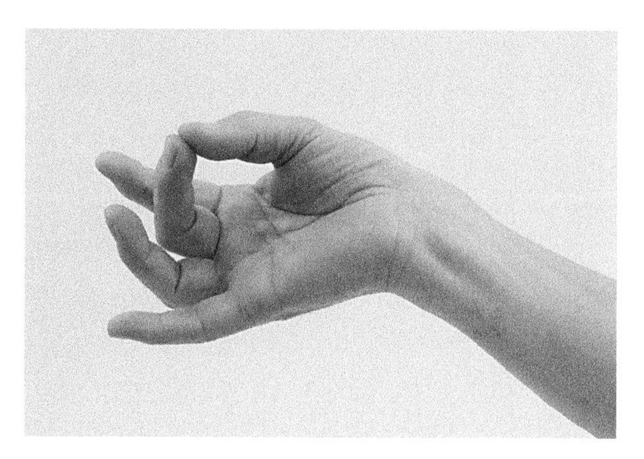

**With each hand:** Create a circle using your thumb and middle finger and hold the hand open. The other fingers are relaxed.

**Effect:** Strengthens digestive power (Agni); calms the mind for meditation and improves concentration and contemplation (Prana); eases muscle spasms, especially in the jaw muscles; strengthens Pitta (because the middle finger is the Pitta finger).

**Marmas that are involved and strengthened:** Sthapani (tip of the thumb), Talahridaya (in the confluence of the energy pathways of the middle finger and thumb), Kurcha and Kurchashira (slight tension in the ball of the thumb).

**Practice time:** 5–10 minutes twice daily.

## Life or Prana Mudra

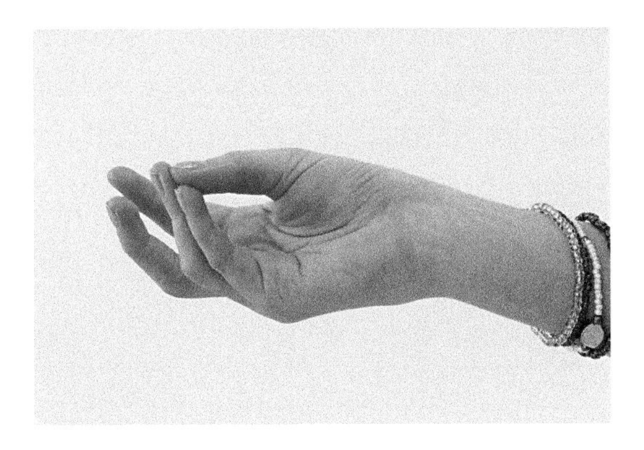

**With each hand:** Place thumb, little finger and ring finger together to form a circle, letting the other fingers relax and stretch out.

**Effect:** The energies in the root Chakra and sexual Chakra as well as Guda and Basti Marma are strengthened. This has a rejuvenating effect on the reproductive tissue (Shukra). Eyesight (Alochaka) improves; vitality (Bala, Ojas) and joy in life increase. Guiding Prana to the heavy elements – water (ring finger) and earth (little finger) – has the effect of grounding excess mental activity and settles thinking when there is too much Vata in the nervous system.

**Marmas that are involved and strengthened:** Talahridaya (in the confluence of the energy pathways of the little finger, ring finger and thumb), Kurcha and Kurchashira (slight tension in the ball of the thumb), Guda and Basti (elements of earth and water) since the little finger and ring finger are involved and the root of the thumb (Guda and Basti) is contracted.

**Practice time:** 5–10 minutes twice daily.

## Mudra for orientation

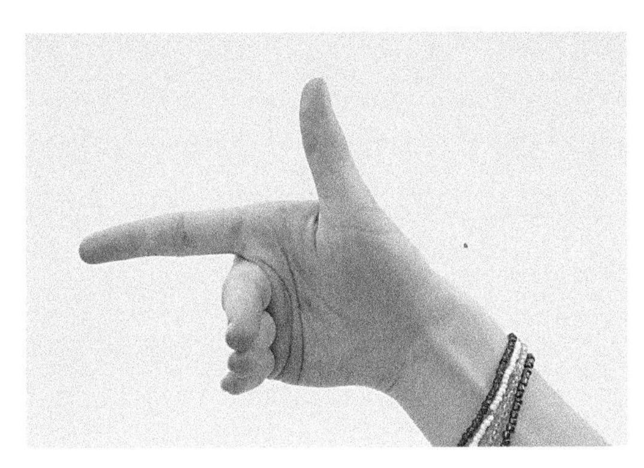

**With each hand:** Stretch your index finger forward and the thumb up, stretching your other fingers at a right angle. The hand now projects the three directions in space.

**Effect:** Promotes mental relaxation and concentration (Prana); directs the consciousness (Sadhaka); strengthens the back (Avalambaka); gives vitality (Ojas, Bala); helps you find your way.

**Marmas that are involved and strengthened:** Ani (index finger stretched, reflexology zone on the back of the finger), Lohitaksha (corresponding area in the stretched crease between the thumb and the forefinger).

**Practice time:** 5 minutes twice daily.

## The conch shell

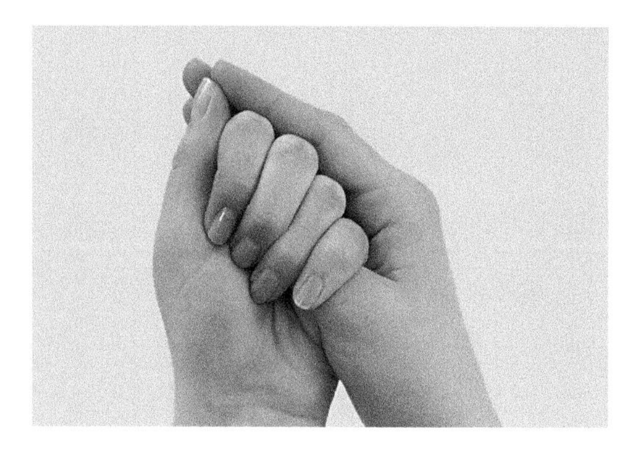

Grasp the right thumb with your left hand and touch the tip of the left thumb with your right index finger.

**Effect:** Supports the treatment of thyroid disorders, hoarse voice, throat inflammation and tonsillitis (Udana), digestive weakness and gastrointestinal disorders (Agni); strengthens the reproductive tissue (Shukra) and gives peace to the heart (Sadhaka).

**Marmas that are involved and strengthened:** Talahridaya and all Kshipras of the left hand, Kurcha (left hand), Kurchashira (right hand).

**Practice time:** 5–10 minutes twice daily.

## Vayu Mudra

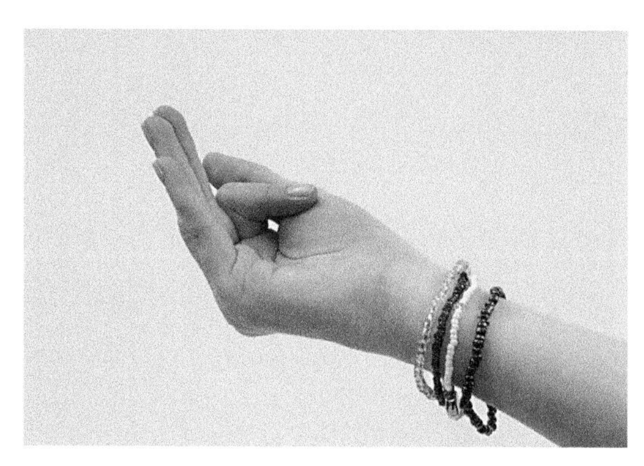

**With each hand:** Bend your index finger and lay it parallel to the thumb on the ball of the thumb. The other fingers are together and stretched; the hand is opened upward.

**Effect:** The wind of Vata (air element) sits in the index finger, which is bound to the thumb and is soothed. This Mudra calms Vata beautifully and relaxes it mainly in its root (Apana). It warms the abdomen, strengthens digestive fire and harmonizes peristaltic movement (Samana); strengthens the neck, throat, airways (Udana) and the back (Avalambaka); promotes concentration and meditation (Prana); strengthens eyesight (Alochaka).

**Marmas that are involved and strengthened:** Kurcha (adjoining finger), Kshipra (integrated by the locking of the index finger and the thumb), Nabhi (hollow of the palm that accumulates Prana).

**Practice time:** 5–10 minutes twice daily.

## Victory Mudra

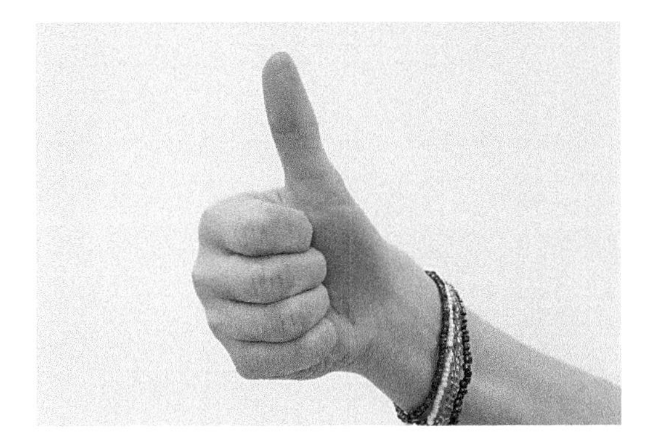

**With each hand:** Form a very narrow fist and stretch your thumb upwards, as in a 'thumbs up' sign.

**Effect:** Gives strength and enthusiasm (Ojas, Bala), joy in the heart, happiness and confidence (Sadhaka); strengthens the back (Avalambaka); calms anxiety (Prana); provides general warming (Agni).

**Marmas that are involved and strengthened:** Brihati and Amsaphalaka (upright thumb; equivalents of these Marmas on the back of the thumb), Talahridaya (fingers into the palm), Ani (equivalent on the back of the index finger), Krikatika (equivalent on the back of the stretched distal phalanx of the thumb).

**Practice time:** 5–10 minutes twice daily.

## The fist

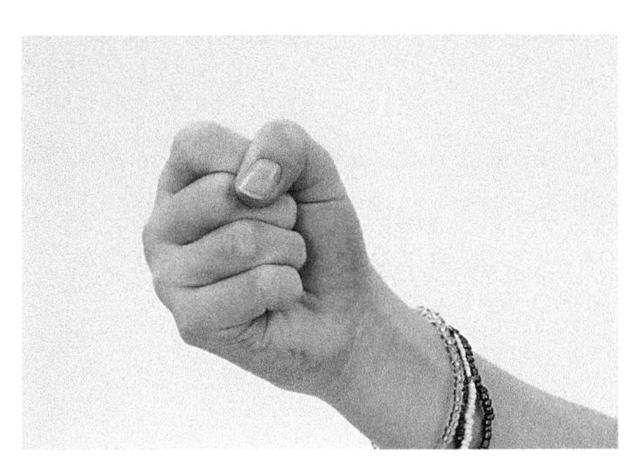

**With each hand:** Form both hands into a loose fist, with thumbs on the outside in front of the middle finger. The fists are in the groin. Sit comfortably upright, close your eyes and feel the energy emanating from the Mudra.

**Effect:** This is one of the best Mudras for strengthening the root Chakra and the Marmas in the pelvic area and in the groin. The fist awakens vitality and *joie de vivre*, stimulates the respiratory system, enlivens Prana in the whole organism and increases energy in the throat Chakra.

**Marmas that are involved and strengthened:** Guda, Lohitaksha, Vitapa, Nabhi and the Marmas of the lower back, especially Kukundara. The vital forces of the lower energy centres are bound and held in the clenched fist. If we put them in the groin, we place them at the root of the body. Shringataka, Nila and Manya will also be strongly affected (on the inside of the distal phalanx of the thumb that touches the back of the middle finger, which has a Pitta quality).

**Practice time:** 5–10 minutes twice daily.

## Coming back to the Self

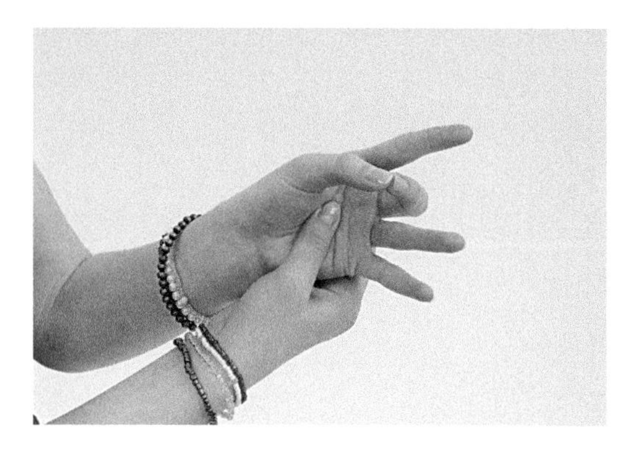

Hold your left hand so that the tip of your right thumb lies in the centre of the left palm. The other fingers lie protectively flat on the back of the hand. The left thumb and middle finger touch each other and form a ring. The fingers that are not involved are stretched and relaxed.

**Effect:** Gives your heart rest, leads back to the Self (Atma), generally relaxes (Prana, Sadhaka) and regenerates; strengthens the solar plexus (Agni, Samana).

**Marmas that are involved and strengthened:** Talahridaya (the tip of the thumb corresponding to the brain rests in the heart of the hand: Prana of thinking is brought back to the Self). From Talahridaya all the Marmas of the hand are nourished and strengthened. The middle finger (Pitta) resting on the thumb upholds the dynamic and transformative power of Pitta for regeneration.

**Practice time:** 5–10 minutes twice daily.

## Mudra for self-confidence

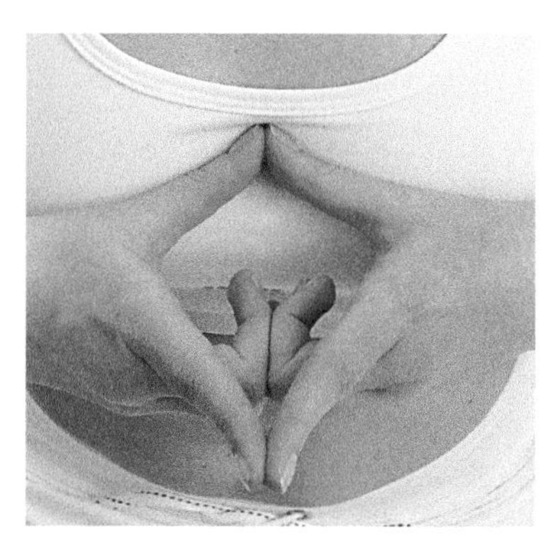

Place the tips of the thumb and index fingers so that, when viewed from above, they appear to form a bow and arrow. With the other three fingers bent at a right angle, bring them together so that they touch (see photo above). You can bend the bow by stretching your thumb towards yourself. Your index fingers face forward like an arrow. Make sure that the other three fingers are touching, as explained above. Now move the thumb tips along your sternum, searching for a particularly sensitive point or area. You will feel it when you move slowly up and down in the lower third of the sternum. Place your thumbs here: it is a specific point in the heart Marma where condensed emotions are stored. Sit upright and breathe gently and naturally.

**Effect:** As the name implies, this Mudra strengthens self-confidence. It touches the feelings of the heart and awakens joy (Sadhaka); it also strengthens the back (Avalambaka).

**Marmas that are involved and strengthened:** Hridaya (direct contact), Brihati (its counterpart on the back), Amsaphalaka (enlivenment of protective mechanisms on the back).

**Practice time:** 5–10 minutes twice daily.

# Yoga and Marmas

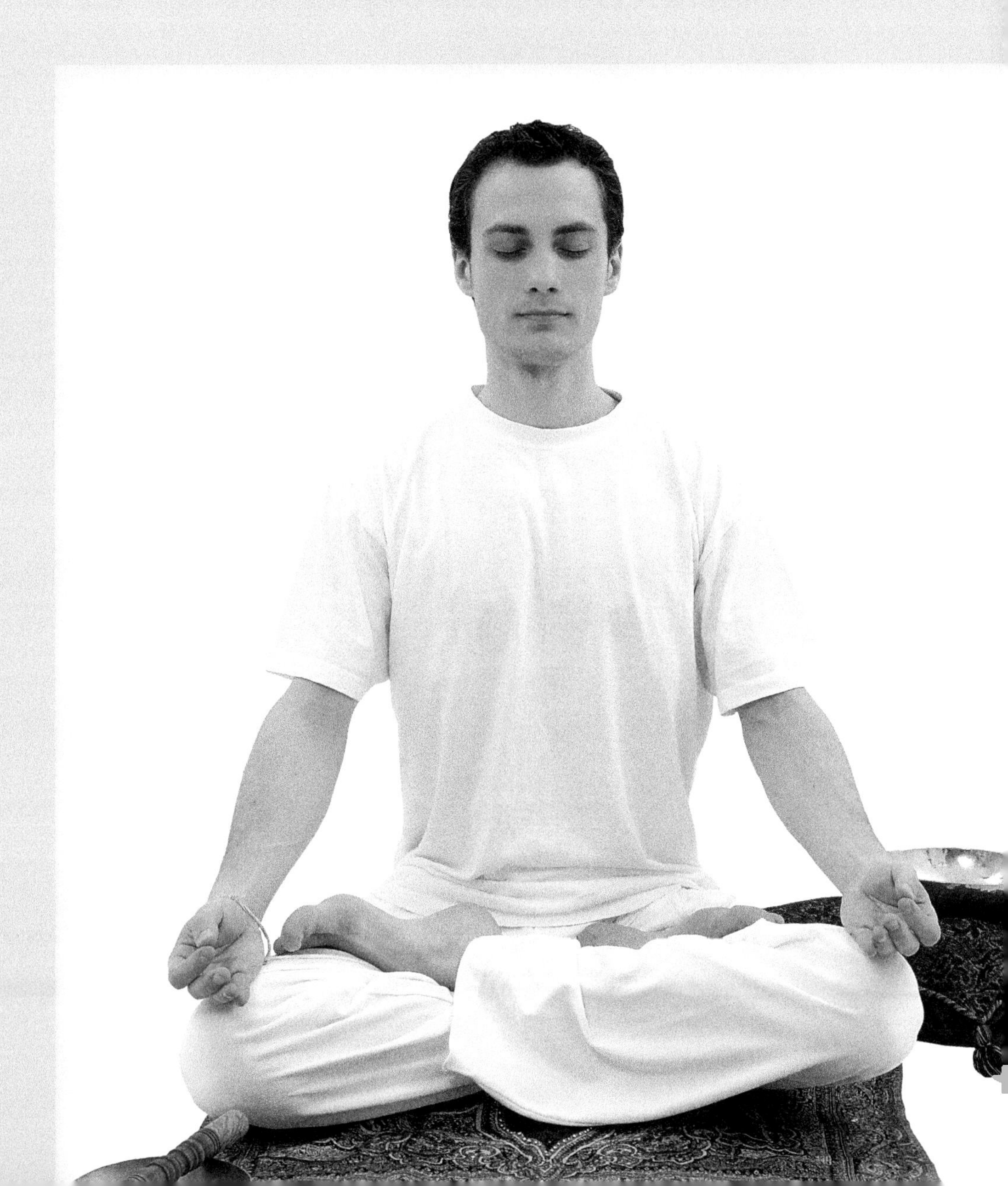

# Strengthening the Marmas with Properly Executed Yoga Asanas

**'Yoga is that state of consciousness where the mind comes to silence. Then the seer experiences his own nature. Otherwise, its true nature is overshadowed by the activity of the mind.'**

MAHARISHI PATANJALI, *YOGA SUTRAS* 2–4

Yoga is a philosophical system that has been in existence for many thousands of years and, like Ayurveda, originates from the Veda. Today, especially in the West, it is known for the physical exercises. However, Yoga is a comprehensive approach to self-discovery and includes behaviour, nutrition, ethics and morality and, above all, meditation. Through meditation, the mental approach of Yoga, that is, by using the mind, we experience rest in the body as well as silence in consciousness. Through the physical exercises of the Yoga system, the Asanas, we experience rest and coherence through physical means, while simultaneously experiencing silence in the mind. The path of Yoga leads to the Self, the Atma, the basis of all Marmas. Through Yoga we comprehensively harmonize and strengthen the system of Marmas. In this way Yoga keeps us young and fit, gives us new energy and refines our perception of the energies of our mind and body and the silent intelligence that underlies nature and the cosmos.

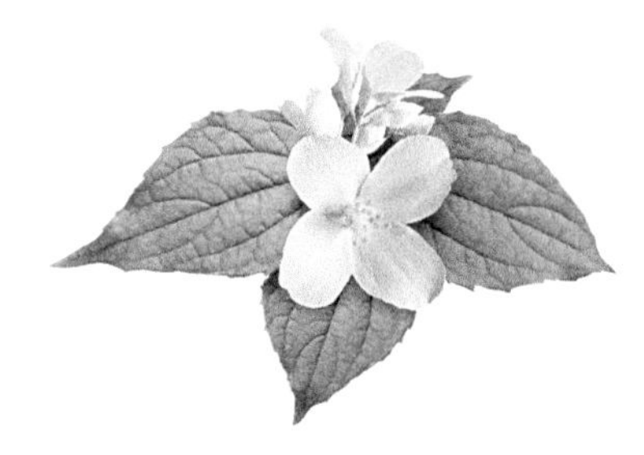

### THE BEST TIME FOR YOGA

The best time for Yoga is when you have some peace and quiet for the practice. The best time is in the morning before breakfast or in the evening before dinner.

There are different schools of Yoga, which often have quite different views on the selection of Asanas, the nature of their execution and the aim of the exercises. The proper exercise of the Asanas stimulates, opens and strengthens different Marmas, depending on the body posture and movement. Marmas are like batteries – they become charged by Yoga postures and movements that are performed correctly. With smooth, flowing movement, gentle stretching and finally the restful position at the end of each Asana, the natural flow of energy is supported in the subtle energy channels of the body, the Nadis.

## Yoga is not gymnastics

It is not about achieving certain end positions that appear in books. The goal of Yoga is not acrobatics, but to create order and stillness in mind and body. The first mistake you can make – and this is a very common mistake, which is even taught by some Yoga teachers in their classes – is to force yourself into the end position, with strenuous stretching. This will only prevent the desired effect from occurring. The desired effect is to open the Marmas and charge them with energy. Painful stretching stops this from happening – and it may also cause injury.

## Your well-being is the measure of success

The path is this: move slowly and easily towards the desired final position of an Asana. Just when you have reached the point at which the greatest comfort ceases, remain in this position, no matter how far you may still be from the theoretically defined end posture. The only important thing is: it must feel so good that you do not want to leave that position, and in this way it will be doing you good. So stay inwardly focused and enjoy the relaxation and the increasing energy. It flows into the opened and gently stretched Marmas or their corresponding points. Always breathe naturally, evenly and steadily. Make sure all the movements are done smoothly, slowly and from a state of inner settledness and peace. Avoid sudden movements!

## Remain relaxed throughout

If you are a beginner and are learning the Asanas for the first time, then do not pay attention to every detail of each posture but make sure that you do not involuntarily hold your breath. Do not worry about practising the Asana perfectly – just take it easy and start. After a few days, when you become familiar with the process, gradually begin to coordinate your Asanas with the breathing. If you do it right, then you will notice that your inward and outward breathing will initiate the outward and inward movement of the Asanas.

# The Effect of Yoga Postures on the Marmas

In this section we describe how the Asanas strengthen and charge the Marmas through the example of three typical Yoga postures. Then we recommend a complete yet simple practice set that includes all the Marmas and that, when practised daily, will recharge your energy batteries and preserve health, flexibility and fitness. There are many good Yoga books on the market in which the execution of these particular Asanas is shown step by step in pictures and text (see Van Lysebeth and Congreve 2000 in Further Reading and Useful Addresses). If necessary, you could also contact a Yoga teacher.

## Diamond posture – Vajrasana

The diamond posture (see illustrations on page 124) increases self-confidence and strengthens the back, clarifies the mind and opens the chest and the breathing. It reduces tension in the extensor muscles of the legs and facilitates the flow of energy in the Nadis of the spine up to the head Marmas. Gulpha, the ankle Marma on the foot, is opened by the stretch and stimulated by the gentle pressure of the weight of the body. The counterpoint of Indrabasti on the extensor side of the lower leg is also stretched and opened, as also is the knee Marma. The Talahridaya of the hand is on the Ani Marma on the thigh; it strengthens and soothes it, and in addition the stretching of the knee also opens Ani. The energy in the spinal cord Nadis Ida, Pingala and Sushumna can flow freely.

## Sitting forward bend – Janu Sirasana

The forward bend (see illustrations on page 124) stretches and relaxes the lower back, which makes energy flow into the pelvic area and especially into the root Chakra and Guda Marma. In the movement sequence all the back Marmas are opened from bottom to top. In the restful end position the Sushumna energy flows upwards and collects in the pituitary gland and in the third eye, that is, in Sthapani. Guda is addressed by the pressure of the heel and the Marmas of the lower back by the stretching. It is also a beneficial exercise for Brihati, which is gently stretched and charged. The physical contact with Janu Marma has a soothing effect on Sthapani and promotes inner silence and concentration in the resting position.

## Half spinal twist – Matsyendrasana

The rotation of the spine and the stretching of all the muscles of the trunk activate all the Marmas of the back, abdomen and chest and, in addition, the Marmas of the arm, Manibandha, Indrabasti, Kurpara, Ani, Urvi, Lohitaksha and Kakshadhara are involved when the arm supports the posture. The half spinal twist (see illustration on page 125) promotes elasticity of the spine and prevents sciatica and muscular discomfort in the legs. Internal organs such as the liver, pancreas, spleen, bladder, kidneys and adrenals are compressed and massaged and blood flow increases.

## A simple practice set for all Marmas

### 1. Becoming aware of oneself

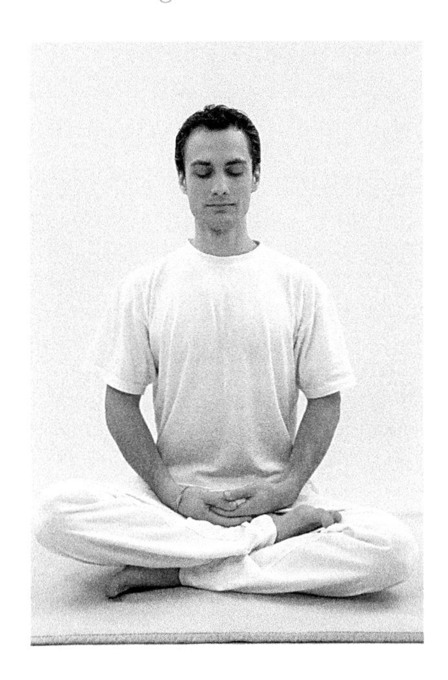

Bringing the attention back to the body has a calming and balancing effect on all the Marmas and stimulates the flow of energy in the Nadis. Sit comfortably, direct your attention inwards and let your body and mind come to rest.

### 3. Rolling – Vellan

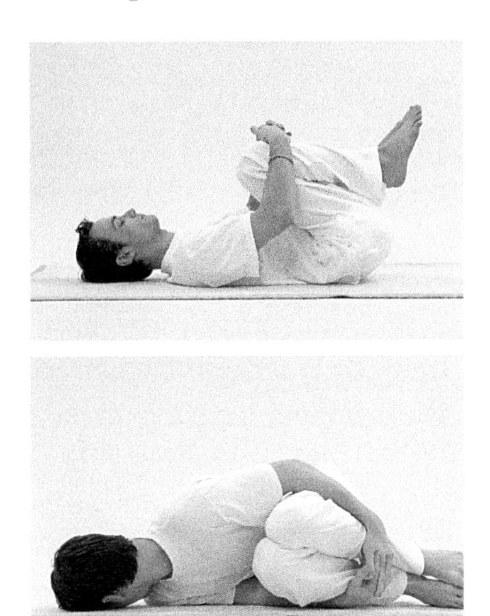

Vellan is relaxing and loosening, especially on the Marmas of the spine and shoulders and on the muscles of the back. Hold your knees with clasped hands and breathe in. As you exhale, slowly roll to the side and stay there for a moment. As you then inhale, roll back; then exhale and roll to the other side.

### 2. Enlivening exercise – Samvahana

The hands and their Marmas come into physical contact with the entire body and bring lymphatic and other fluids and energies to the heart. Almost all the Marmas are gently massaged. The hands always keep in contact with the body and massage through pressing and sliding along the body – in a gentle kneading movement – in the direction of the heart. Start at the forehead and face and proceed as shown in the illustrations.

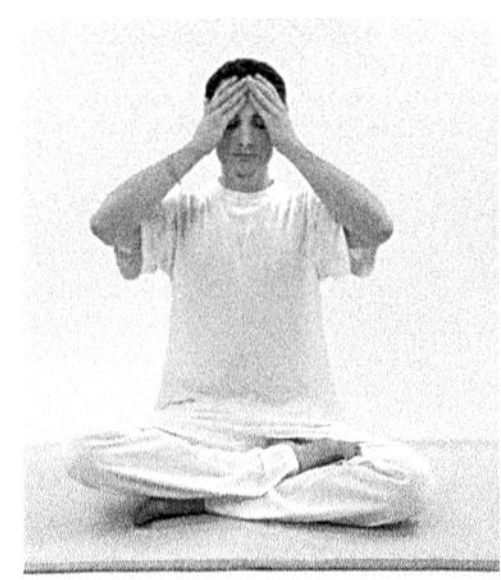
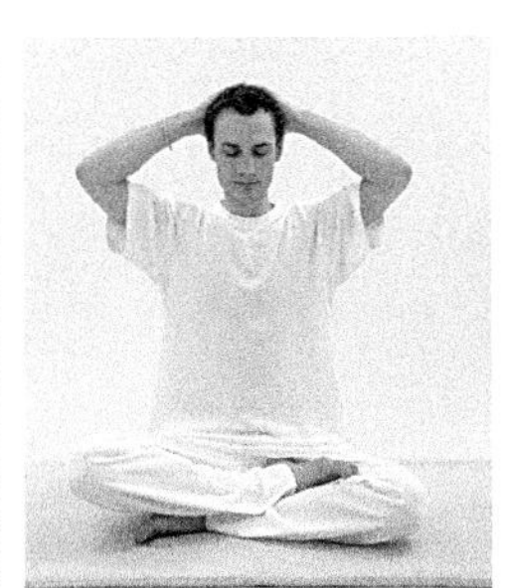
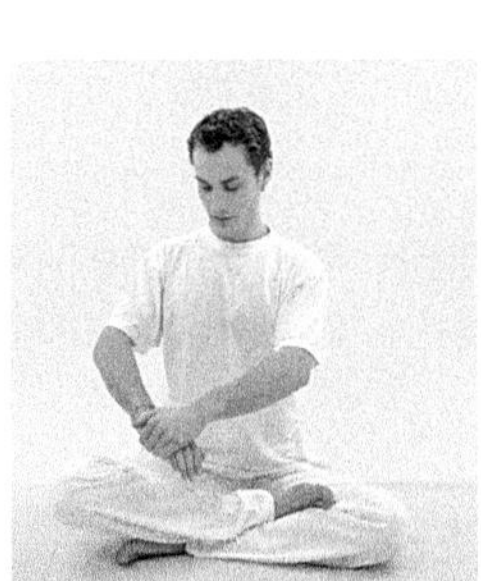
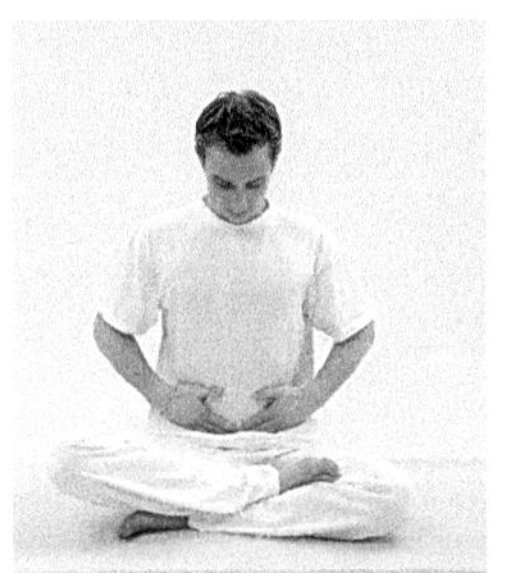
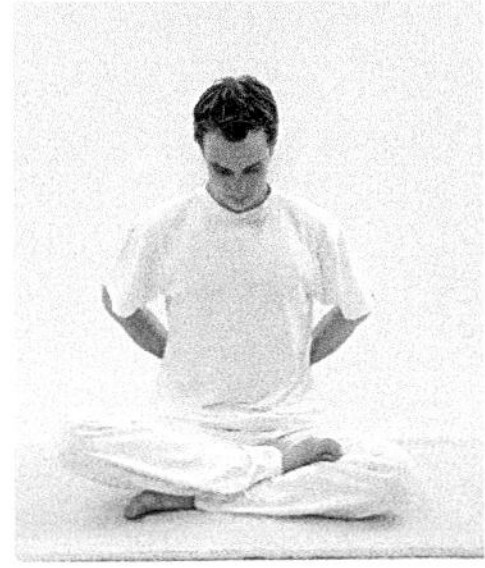
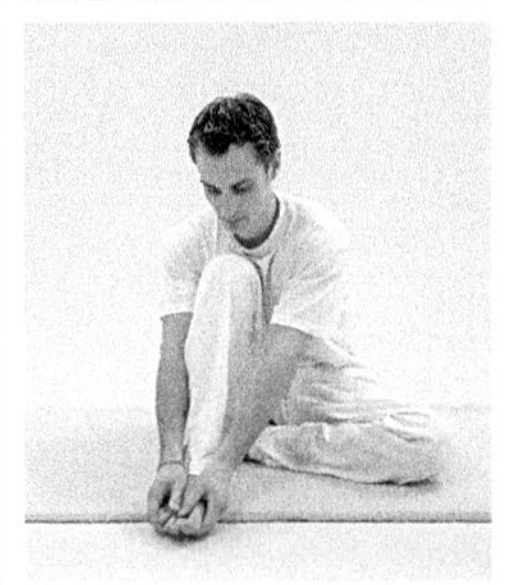

## 4. Diamond posture – Vajrasana

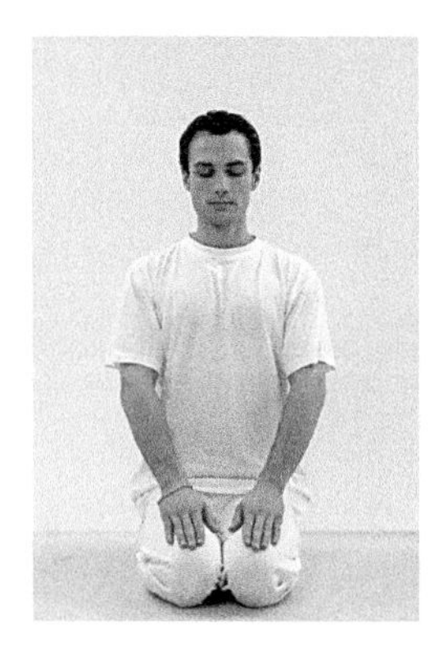

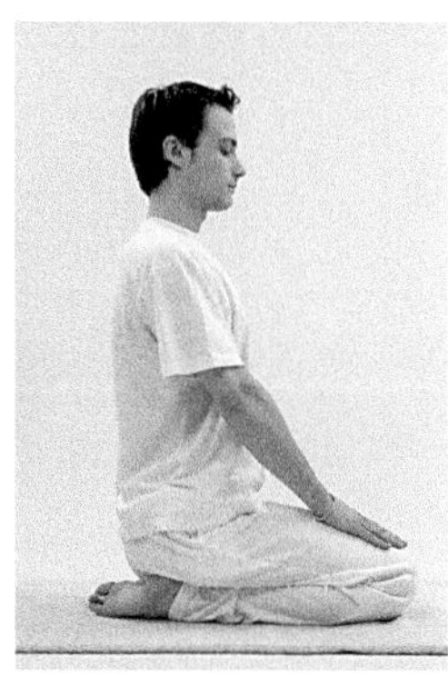

The diamond posture increases self-confidence and strengthens the back, clarifies the mind and opens the chest and the breathing; it also opens Gulpha and other Marmas.

## 5. The forward bend – Janu Sirasana

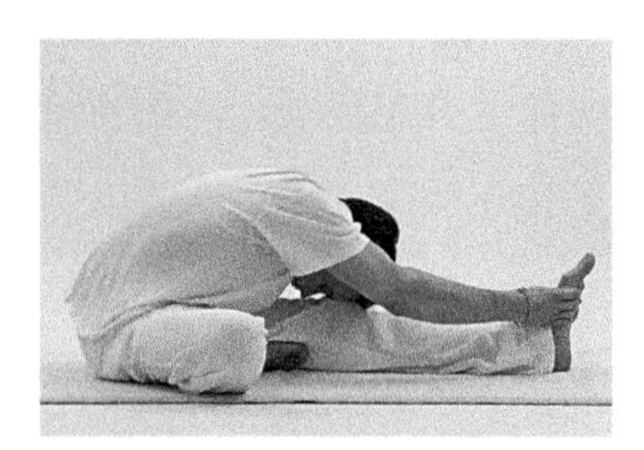

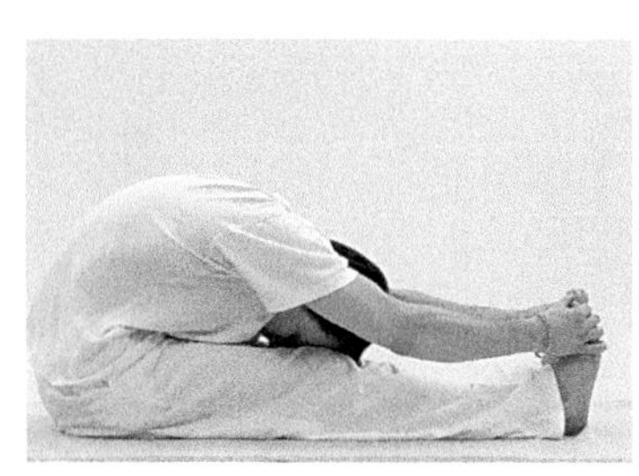

The forward bend stretches and relaxes the lower back, resulting in more energy in the pelvic area and especially in the root Chakra and Guda. All back Marmas are opened.

## 6. Shoulder stand – Sarvangasana

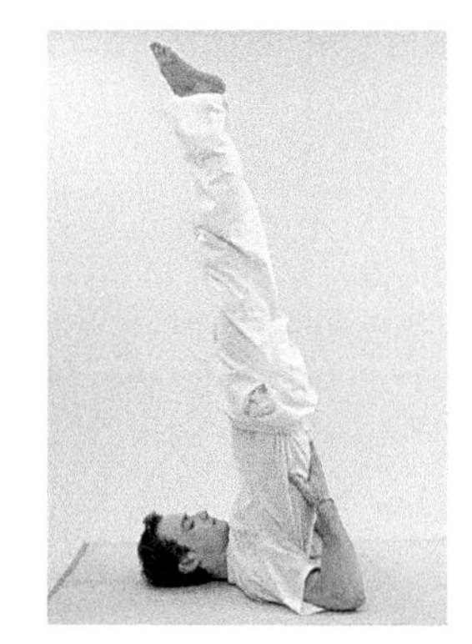

By compressing the anterior neck region and increasing blood pressure in the head, the neck and head Marmas are particularly stimulated, Adhipati and Simanta included.

## 7. Cobra – Bhujangasana

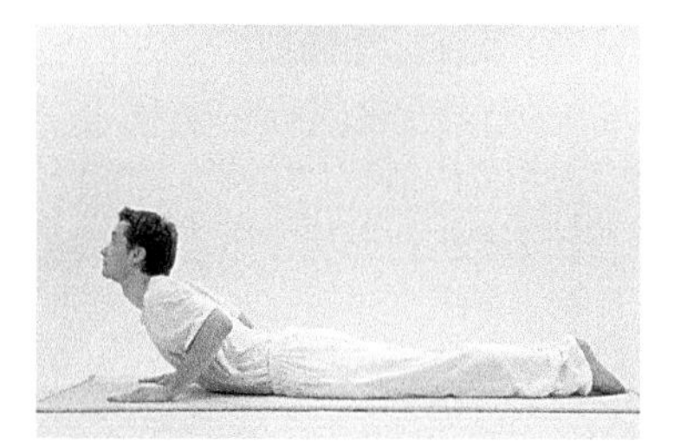

The stretching of the neck opens the throat Marmas, and the expansion of the chest opens Hridaya and the other chest Marmas. The lumbar and gluteal muscles are contracted and therefore the Marmas in this region are stimulated.

8. Locust – Shalabhasana

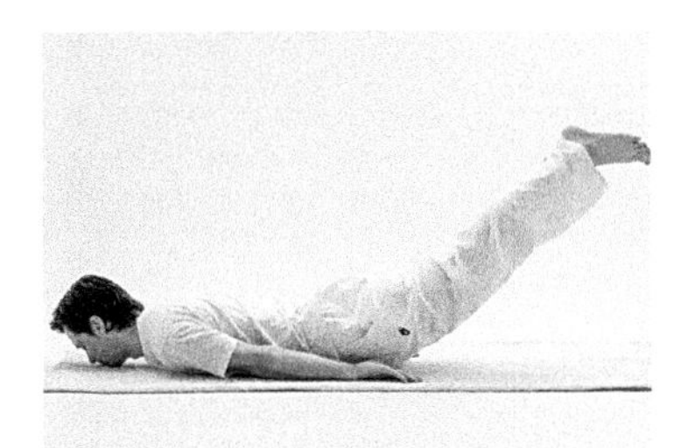

In the locust posture the Lohitaksha and Vitapa Marmas are opened and vitalized by the stretching in the groin area. The tension in the buttocks and the lumbar muscles stimulates all the Marmas of the pelvis and lower back.

9. Bow – Dhanurasana

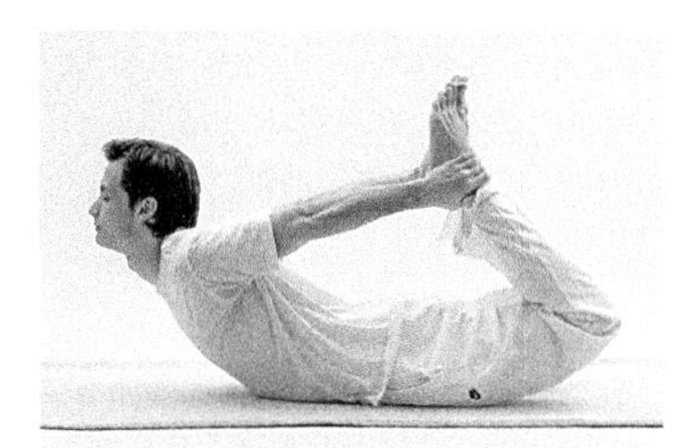

In this Asana, the groin Marmas Lohitaksha and Vitapa, in particular, are stretched and freed of tension. Also, the ankle Marma Gulpha and the thigh Marmas are opened. In contrast, the Marmas of the whole back are strengthened by the muscular tension and the position of the spine, while the Marmas of the chest are enlivened through the stretch. The abdominal Marmas are stimulated by the rolling on the floor.

10. Half spinal twist – Matsyendrasana

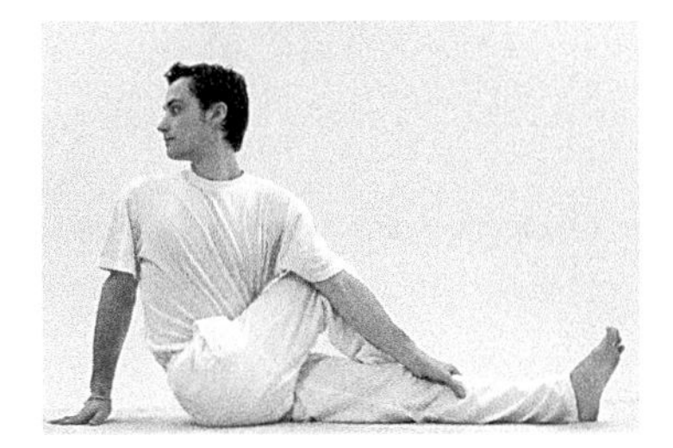

The rotation of the spine and the stretching of all the muscles of the trunk massages the internal organs and stimulates all the Marmas of the back, abdomen and chest, as well as the various Marmas of the supporting arm.

11. Standing forward bend – Uttanasana

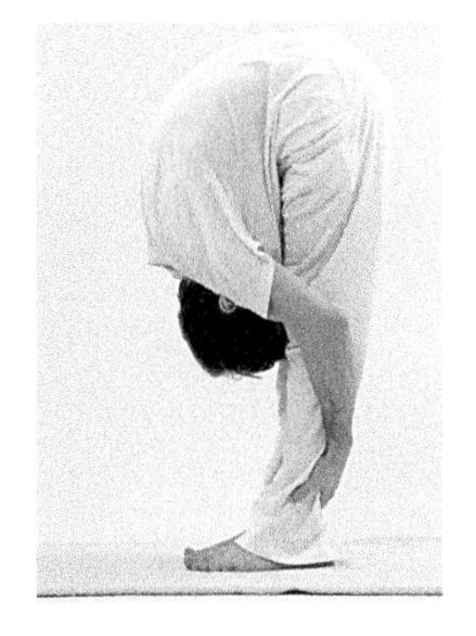

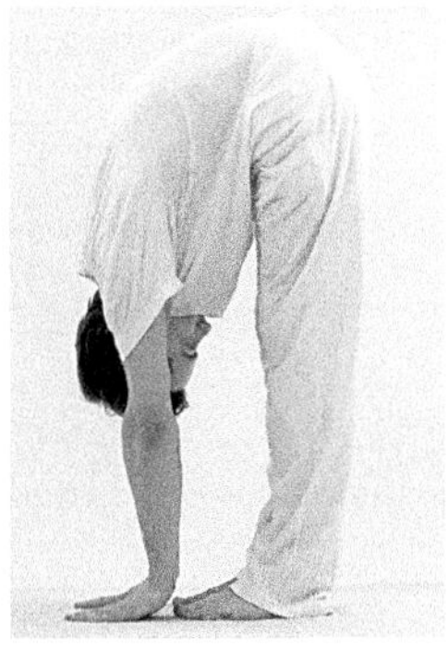

The increased blood flow to the head addresses all the head Marmas, and all the back Marmas are stretched and opened.

### 12. Resting position – Savasana

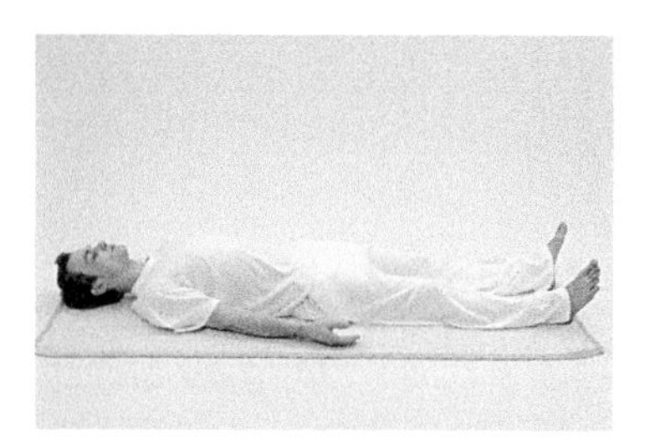

The previous exercises set regeneration and healing processes in motion for the whole body. The organism now needs some minutes of complete relaxation and peace to bring this process to completion. Numerous Marmas were touched, opened, compressed or stimulated and their inner intelligence enlivened. Savasana balances all the Marmas and charges them with new energy.

## Pranayama – gentle alternate nostril breathing

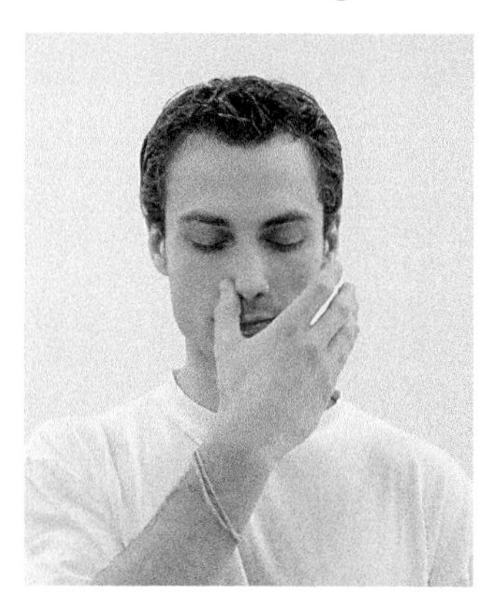

This simple and natural breathing exercise calms the body, harmonizes the nervous system and nourishes the body and its Marmas with Prana. It is called Sukha Pranayama – easy breathing – and creates balance between the left and right hemispheres of the brain, and in this way coordinates the different functions of body and mind. It is a particularly effective technique to treat Phana, the nose Marma, with its two main points left and right of the nostrils. Phana controls the sense of smell, Kapha in the head area and the mucous membranes of the nose and sinuses. Through Pranayama we revitalize this Marma and bring Prana to all other energy channels and Marmas. Also, with Ayurvedic Nasya Therapy, an application of oil or ghee to the nasal mucosa, we can act from the inside on this Marma. We can also combine this local application with Pranayama, by applying some Ayurvedic oil inside the nose before starting the breathing exercise. Pranayama is a good preparation for meditation, because it draws attention inside and calms the breathing. When you do Pranayama, you may notice a pleasant lightness in the body and mental clarity, and also feel the energy in your nervous system recharging.

### How to do Pranayama

Sit upright comfortably and put the thumb of your right hand on the right Phana Marma, above the nasal wing (see photo opposite). Now start the breathing exercise by closing the right nostril with the thumb and breathe out and in through the left nostril. Now close the left nostril with the middle and ring fingers of the right hand and breathe out and in again on the right side. Using this rhythm, always close one nostril at a time during an exhalation and then an inhalation; continue breathing in a natural and relaxed way. Breathe through alternate nostrils in this way for about five minutes. Breathe calmly and evenly; let the breath come and go by itself.

# Marma Therapy for Everyday Complaints

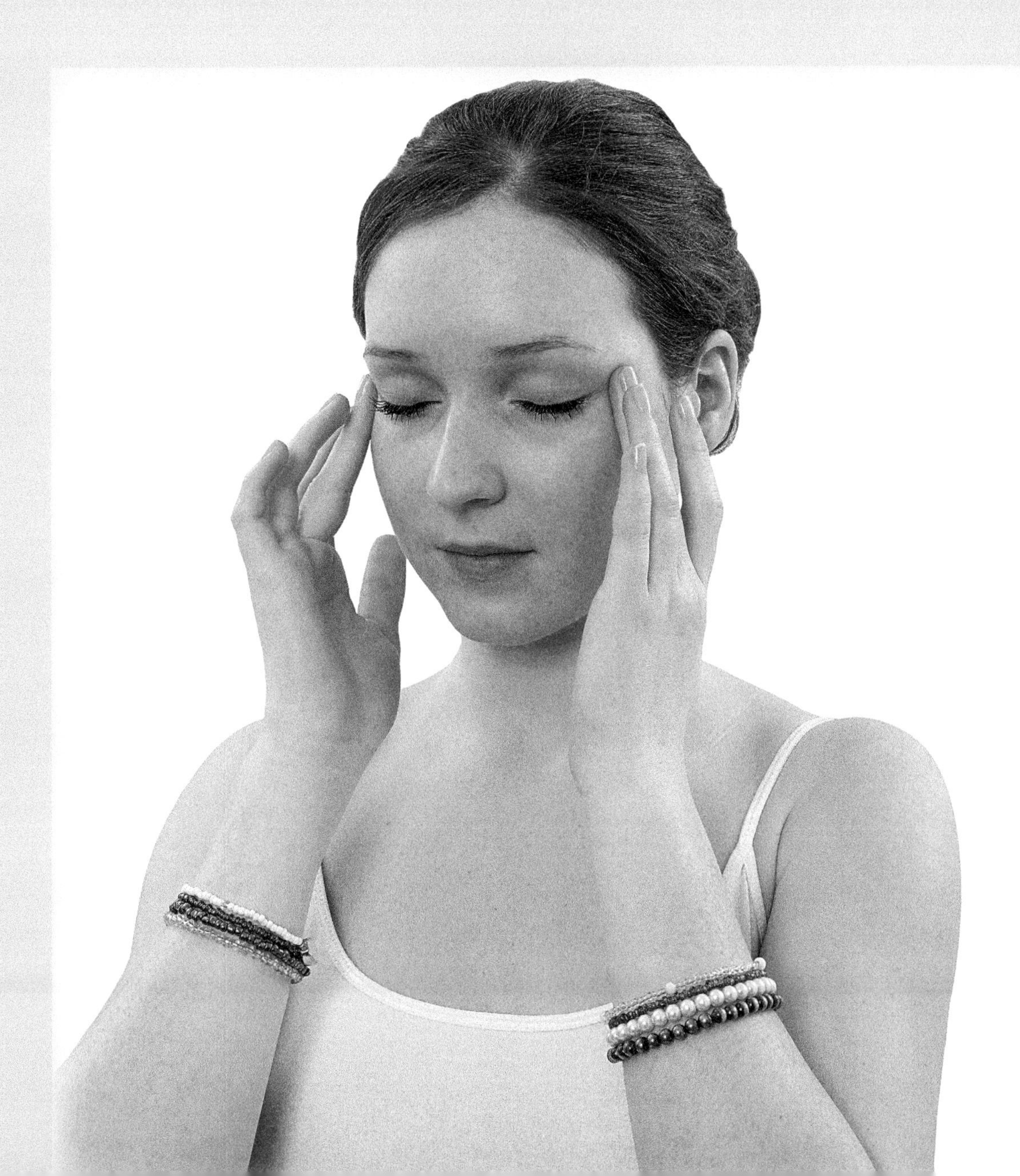

# Supporting Self-healing with Marmas and Ayurveda

Marma treatment is a flexible method that can be used in different ways with various diseases or everyday complaints. Often it is enough to treat a single Marma by simply touching it, applying an oil, massaging it gently, applying a heat pack, irradiating it with colour or light or by applying a suitable ointment. The art of medicine – especially with chronic or deeper disorders – is to combine several Marmas within a treatment properly.

How many Marmas and which ones are included in a treatment naturally depends on the type of physical or mental imbalance. Basically, we can choose Marmas from various aspects:

- One possibility is to treat a central Marma with its peripheral counterparts. So, for example, combine treatment of the Basti Marma over the bladder with the Indrabasti Marmas on the calves and forearms. In bladder weakness, pelvic complaints, gynaecological problems or weakness in the lower back, this combination would be useful.

- We can also choose Marmas according to disturbance in Doshas. Vata disorders like anxiety, sleep disorders or lack of stability can be treated very well with the joint Marmas (Gulpha, Janu, Manibandha, Kurpara) in combination with Adhipati and Simanta.

- An experienced therapist can also integrate the Nadis in his treatment approach, for example by opening and enlivening the channels of breathing and Prana by combining the Kshipra Marmas on the hands with Phana, Hridaya and Brihati.

In this chapter we provide some examples which should give you a feeling of how to perform self or partner treatment for everyday ailments and how to complement the Marma treatment with other Ayurvedic approaches.

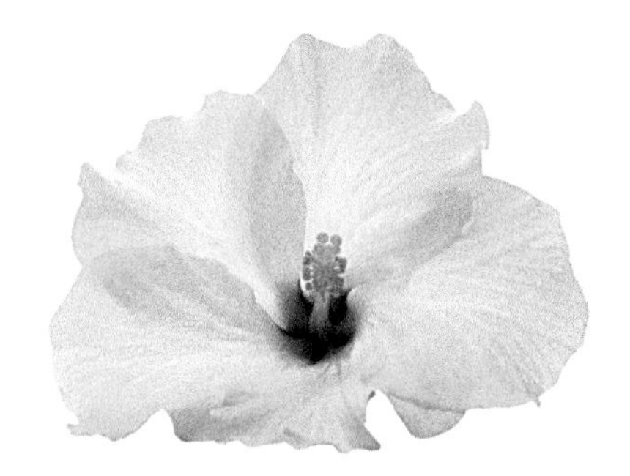

## IMPORTANT POINTS FOR MARMA THERAPY

### Rest, settling down, breathing

Before you begin, take at least 2 to 3 minutes to settle down – maybe even do Pranayama, the gentle alternate nostril breathing exercise (page 126) to strengthen your Prana (this applies both to you and your partner).

### First address the three 'Super-Ministries' or Mahamarmas

For a more detailed treatment and whenever greater healing power is required, first make contact with the three major Marmas of the heart, bladder and head (Sthapani or Adhipati) that rule over all the other Marmas and have the largest energy reservoirs. Even placing the hands on the Mahamarmas will strengthen the effects of treating other Marmas and also makes contact with them. If time and circumstances allow, treat them with an aroma Marma oil.

### First treat the related peripheral Marmas

If you perform an eye treatment, for example, then begin (after making contact with the three major Marmas) with massage of the related peripheral Marmas on the hands and feet and then continue with massage of the points on the head.

### Sequence on arms and legs

If we want to release stress, then the order is from top to bottom and from inside out. So first we treat the Marmas on the arm and then on the leg – starting with the arm and finishing with the hand and similarly starting with the leg and ending with the foot. Conversely, if we want to increase energy and also bring this energy into the central Marmas then we do the opposite. In the examples given below the treatment sequence is specified.

### Please note

Depending on the situation, you may also choose to treat other Marmas than those specified. For the diseases that are listed, medical advice and treatment may be required. We are just giving some suggestions for supporting natural self-healing powers.

## Nervous disorders of the heart

Nervous disorders of the heart, such as undefined feelings of pressure, heart pain due to grief and heart palpitations in response to the slightest excitement, respond very well to Marma treatment.

### The most important Marmas

- Hridaya (pages 76–77): calms and strengthens Prana in the heart
- Sthapani (pages 104–105): in grief, sorrow
- Adhipati (pages 108–109): calms the nervous system
- Nila/Manya (pages 92–93): in palpitations in the heart or in the throat
- Talahridaya, hand (pages 46–47): strengthening of Ojas
- Manibandha (pages 48–49): in heart palpitations
- Kurpara (pages 52–53): calming, for fear
- Talahridaya, feet (pages 58–59): grounding and calming
- Janu (pages 64–65): anxiety
- Basti (pages 72–73): in existential fear

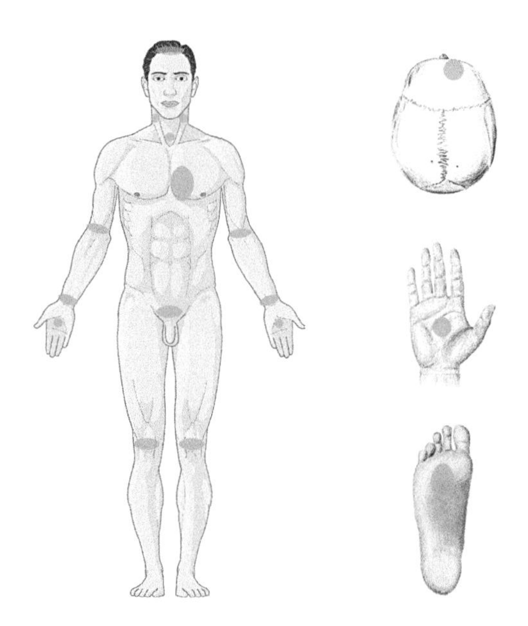

### Oils

- Worry Free oil in almond oil: grief, sorrow
- Vata massage oil: generally relaxing; rose oil: comforts and calms
- Adhimarma: Hridaya, Emotional Relief (Sadhaka)

### Mudras

- Mudra for self-confidence (page 118)
- Anjali Mudra (Hridaya, page 111)

### Breathing exercises and Yoga Asanas

- Pranayama (page 126)
- Becoming aware of oneself (page 123)
- Half spinal twist (page 125)
- Diamond posture (page 124)

### The following are also helpful

- *Gandharva music:* Daily – 10 minutes in the morning and/or at night before bedtime; has a very calming influence on the autonomic nervous system.
- *Raisin water:* Soak a handful of raisins overnight in a glass of water and drink the water in the morning (the raisins can, for example, be used on cereal).
- *Magnesium:* A magnesium deficiency can cause heart rhythm disorders or nervous heart conditions.
- *Meditation:* Meditation and relaxation are effective remedies for nervous disorders of all kinds. Transcendental Meditation has proven to be particularly effective.

## Sleep disorders

Common causes of sleep disorders include overstimulation of the senses, eating a heavy meal in the evening or eating too late, consumption of coffee or black tea and going to bed late (after 10pm the biorhythm of an energy phase begins, making it more difficult to fall asleep).

### The most important Marmas

▶ Adhipati (pages 108–109) and Simanta (pages 106–107): soothe the nervous system

▶ Sthapani (pages 104–105): settles thinking

▶ Talahridaya, feet (pages 58–59): makes you drowsy

▶ Gulpha (pages 60–61): gives inner comfort

▶ Manibandha (pages 48–49): soothes and makes you feel drowsy at night

▶ Nabhi (pages 74–75): centring; strengthens the autonomic nervous system

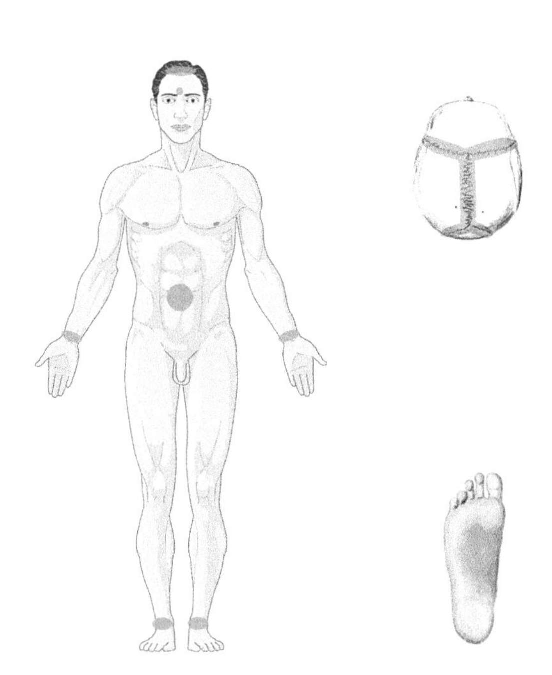

### Oils

▶ Worry Free oil in almond oil or Emotional Relief (Sadhaka) oil: grief, sorrow; ghee: for heat in the legs; Vata massage oil with or without Nidra oil: generally reassuring; valerian, St Johns Wort, lavender: calming and strengthening for the nerves

▶ Adhimarma: Adiprana, Hridaya, Emotional Relief (Sadhaka), Udana

### Mudras

▶ Prana Mudra (page 115), Meditation Mudra (page 114), Mudra on Manibandha (see Manibandha, page 49)

### Breathing exercises and Yoga Asanas

▶ Pranayama (page 126), shoulder stand (page 124)

### The following are also helpful

▶ *Gandharva music:* Daily – 10 minutes in the evening before bedtime; soothes the autonomic nervous system.

▶ *Spiced milk:* Heat up a dash of cinnamon, ginger, cardamom, turmeric and nutmeg in a cup of milk and drink before going to bed.

▶ *Vata tea:* A cup in the evening after dinner calms the mind.

▶ *Meditation:* Meditation (such as Transcendental Meditation) and relaxation are effective for insomnia caused by stress and overwork, nervous tension and shift work.

## Headache and migraine

Headaches can have many causes, which should of course be checked by a doctor. For frequent tension headaches and mild forms of migraine, Marma treatment can often provide quick relief. Rest and relaxation are important – just relaxing for a few minutes and turning your attention inward.

### The most important Marmas

▶ Sthapani (pages 104–105): for excessive focus and concentration

▶ Adhipati (pages 108–109), Simanta (pages 106–107): calm the mind, relax the spirit

▶ Shanka, Utkshepa (pages 100–101): mainly in temporal headache

▶ Avarta, Apanga (pages 94–95): for strained eyes

▶ Nila/Manya, Sira Matrika (pages 92–93): overwork, neck tension

▶ Krikatika (pages 98–99): most important Marma for neck headache

▶ Manibandha (pages 48–49) and Gulpha (pages 60–61): in Vata disorders, nervous overstimulation

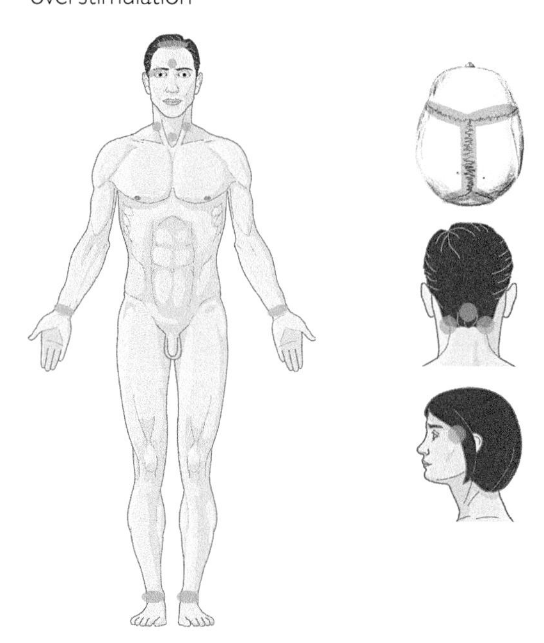

### Oils

▶ Vata massage oil with Vata aroma oil: generally reassuring

▶ Ghee: migraine, temporal headache

▶ Adhimarma: Sthapani, Adhpati, Nila/Manya, Udana

### Yoga, relaxation, meditation

▶ Relaxation exercises, meditation and Yoga reduce stress, relieve tension and headache and prevent migraine.

### The following are also helpful

▶ *MP 16 Nasya oil:* In sinusitis that causes head pressure, inhale 2 or 3 drops repeatedly into the nostrils each day. Also frees from head pressure due to other causes.

▶ *Warm footbath:* At the beginning of a migraine or neck headache.

▶ *Apply sandalwood paste:* Mix sandalwood powder with water or ghee to make a paste and apply on face and/or temples. Helps especially in Pitta headache (desire for cool compress, pounding or throbbing pain).

▶ *Milk compress:* Headache with fever can be alleviated by dipping a washcloth or towel in room-temperature milk, wringing it out and putting it on the forehead. Repeat this several times to divert heat.

## MORE SYMPTOMS AND MARMA COMBINATIONS

Arm and shoulder pain: Amsaphalaka, Amsa, Krikatika, Indrabasti outside and inside (arm), Kurcha and Kurchashira (hand) as point massage and a stroking dissipative massage from the shoulder to the hand

Neck pain: Krikatika, Amsa, Nila/Manya, Sira Matrika, Brihati

Knee pain: Janu, 'The fox head' Mudra (page 65), Ani (leg), Talahridaya (foot), Katikataruna, Nitamba, Kukundara

Restless leg syndrome: Indrabasti (leg), Talahridaya (foot), Gulpha

Abdominal pain: Nabhi, Talahridaya (hand, foot), Kukundara, Parshvasandhi

Menstrual disorders: Basti, Lohitaksha (leg), Parshvasandhi, Kukundara, Urvi and Ani (leg), Gulpha, Talahridaya (foot, hand)

Eye diseases: Talahridaya (foot, hand), Kurcha and Kurchashira (hand), Kshipra between ring finger and little finger, Eye Treatment (pages 94–95)

Anxiety: Sthapani, Adhipati, Simanta, Nila/Manya, Krikatika, Janu, Gulpha, Parshvasandhi, Kurpara (painful tension points at the elbow)

Hoarseness: Nila/Manya, Kshipra (hand), Amsa

Colds, coughs, bronchitis: Hridaya, Brihati, Phana (see page 126), Kshipra (hand)

Skin diseases: Hridaya, Stanarohita, Nabhi, Basti, Talahridaya (hand, foot), Kshipra (feet)

Tinnitus: Sthapani, Nila/Manya, Vidhura, Gulpha, Manibandha, Eye Treatment (pages 94–95), Shringataka

Menopause: Adhipati, Simanta, Eye Treatment (pages 94–95), Nila/Manya, Talahridaya (hand, foot), Shringataka, Phana (page 126), Kukundara, Parshvasandhi, Pranayama (page 126)

Hepatobiliary disorders: Hridaya, Nabhi, Basti, Kshipra and Talahridaya (foot), Janu, Amsa, Brihati

Kidney problems: Kukundara, Parshvasandhi, Gulpha, Indrabasti, Basti, Hridaya

Constipation: Parshvasandhi, Kukundara, Nabhi, Talahridaya (hand, foot), Sthapani

Enuresis in children: Sthapani, Basti, Kukundara, Parshvasandhi, Indrabasti (leg), Talahridaya (feet)

Complete eye treatment: Eye Treatment (pages 94–95) plus: Kurcha right, then left hand, Talahridaya right, then left hand, Kshipra between ring and little finger, right, then left hand, Kurcha right, then left foot, Talahridaya right, then left foot. (This is when treating men – when treating women, left side first, then right.) Then put cotton pads soaked with rose water on the eyes and rest for 5 to 10 minutes.

Menstrual pain: Basti, Lohitaksha (leg), Vitapa, Gulpha, Talahridaya (foot), Kukundara, Parshvasandhi, Sthapani, Nabhi

For self-confidence and courage: Sthapani, Adhipati, Amsa, Hridaya, Brihati, Nabhi, Janu, Gulpha, Hridaya (repeated at the end)

## Complete back treatment

Gentle massage of the back Marmas is mainly suitable for partner treatment and is one of the most comforting Marma applications.

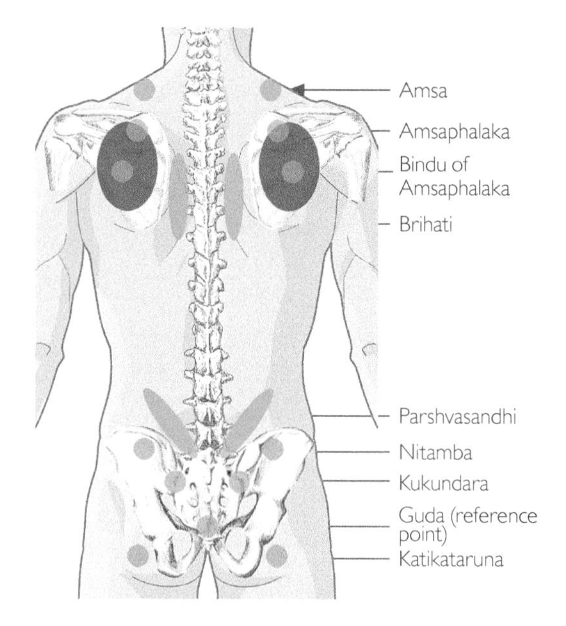


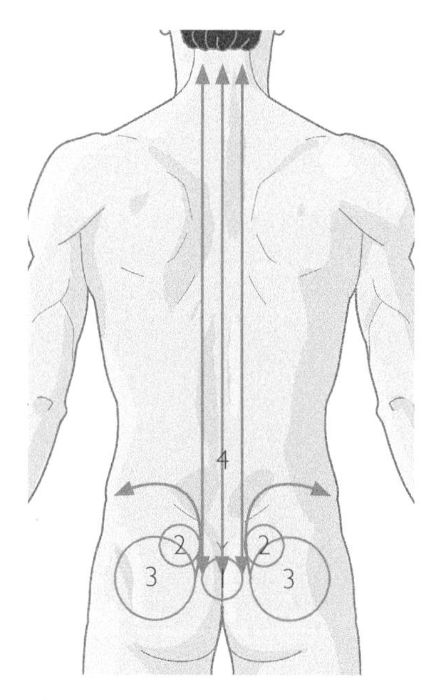


*Massage sequence and procedure*

**Effects:** Relaxes all the muscles of the back, brings the energy channels of the spine – Ida, Pingala and Sushumna – to a gentle flow. Revives and refreshes all the organs of the body, effective against fatigue, back pain, concentration problems, waning memory. Strengthens energy in the spine (Tarpaka, Avalambaka), relaxes the organs of elimination via the reflexology zones and Marmas of the back (Apana), improves digestive power (Pachaka, Ranjaka) and regulates peristalsis (Samana). Loosens the neck shoulder muscles (Udana), calms the heart and circulation (Vyana, Sadhaka) and balances all three Doshas.

**Oils:** For calming and relaxation: Vata massage oil with Vata aroma oil, sesame oil with Vata aroma oil, almond oil, walnut oil; for refreshment: lemongrass, pine, lemon, orange (diluted in almond oil)

**Adhimarma:** Sushumna, Guda, Shanti Om, all in almond oil.

**Treatment time:** 15 to 20 minutes.

### Partner treatment

Your partner lies comfortably and relaxed on the stomach, preferably on a massage table. You stand on their left. First apply oil in the middle of the spine and on the sacrum, lower back and the upper part of the buttocks.

**Treatment format for each massage segment:** 3 times for points 1 to 3 and 7 times for point 4 (see page 34); repeat 2 to 4 times.

**Contact:** The left hand is placed over Brihati Marma in the middle of the thoracic spine, with the right hand over the sacrum.

1. Circular massage with the fingers on the sacroiliac joints

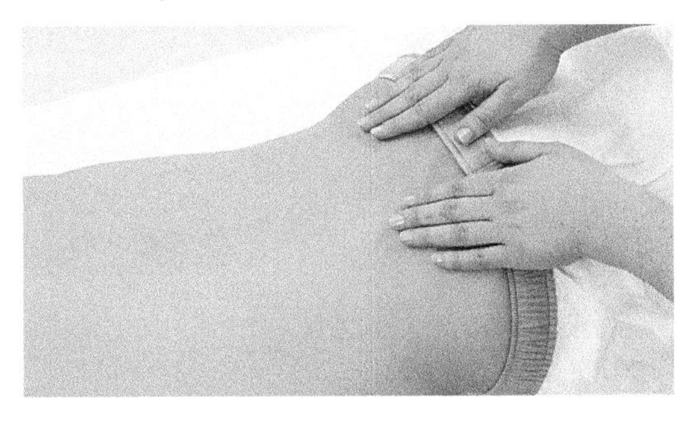

Using the flat of the fingers, massage simultaneously and symmetrically over both sacroiliac joints and the dimples of Venus (spina iliaca posterior superior), the location of Kukundara Marma.

2. Massage of the kidney area and the buttocks

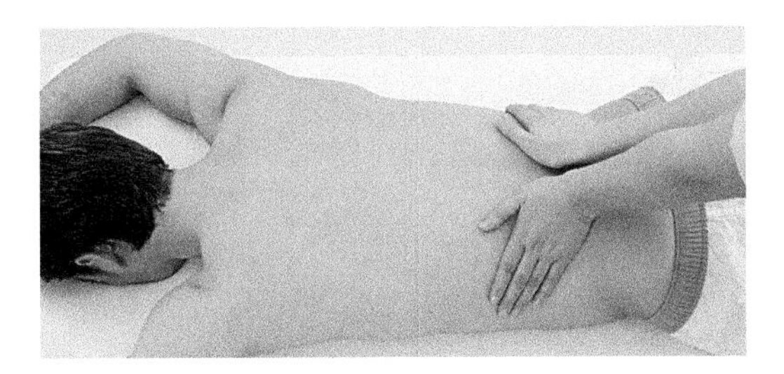

Now we continue with the massage of Parshvasandhi. The seat of this Marma is to the left and right of the lumbar spine, at the transition to the sacrum, and extends in its effect and extent up to the flank, below the bottom rib. Massage up to the kidneys, which are included in the massage of the flanks.

Next we massage with somewhat larger strokes: massage a slightly larger area firstly over the top outer part of the buttocks (Nitamba) and then the central part of the buttocks (Katikataruna).

3. Massage the sacrum with the flat of the hand

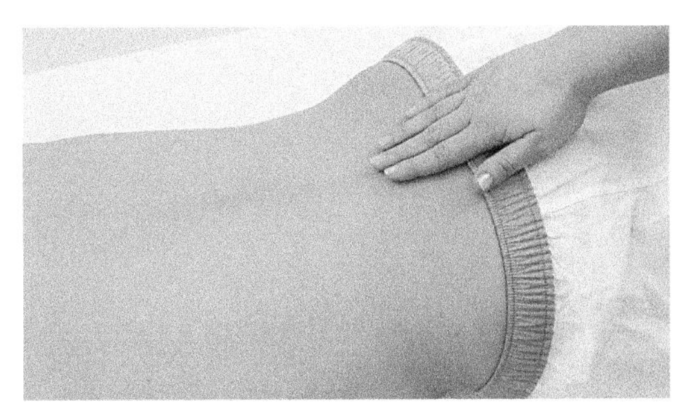

Make gentle clockwise circular motions. Here you also treat the reference point for Guda Marma. It is at the lower end of the sacrum.

Now repeat the massage of the sacrum with the flat of the hand, as described in point 1.

4. Longitudinal strokes along the entire spine

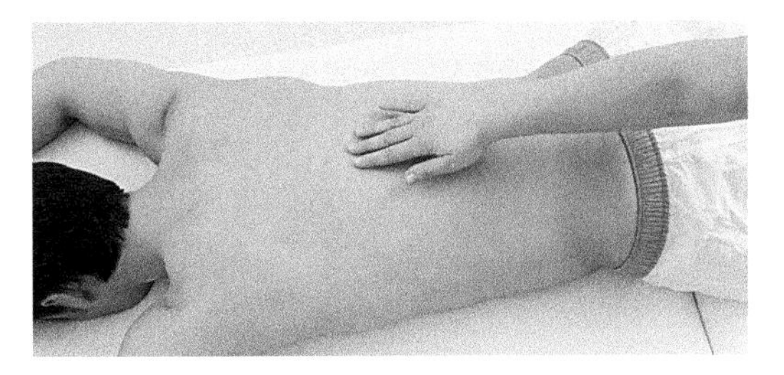

Lay the index, middle and ring fingers of the right hand so that the middle finger is just over the spinous processes in the middle of the spine with the index finger to the left and the ring finger to the right. Starting from the sacrum, move your hand slowly along the spine and then up the neck to the top of the spine at the back of the head. Now move the hand back down the spine, a little faster and with lighter pressure. After every up-and-down stroke let your hand rest on the sacrum for about 10 seconds. Repeat the process 7 times. This treatment includes Parshvasandhi, Brihati, Amsaphalaka, Amsa and Krikatika.

**Completion of treatment:** After the longitudinal strokes repeat points 1 to 3 and end with the hand resting on the sacrum.

## Treatment of the upper back

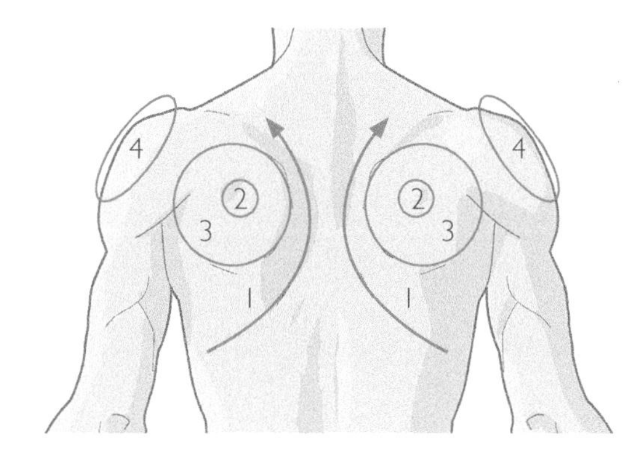


*Massage sequence and procedure*

You can complement the lower back treatment by massaging the upper back, treating the following Marmas: Brihati, Amsaphalaka and Amsa (as described on pages 84–89).

### Self-treatment

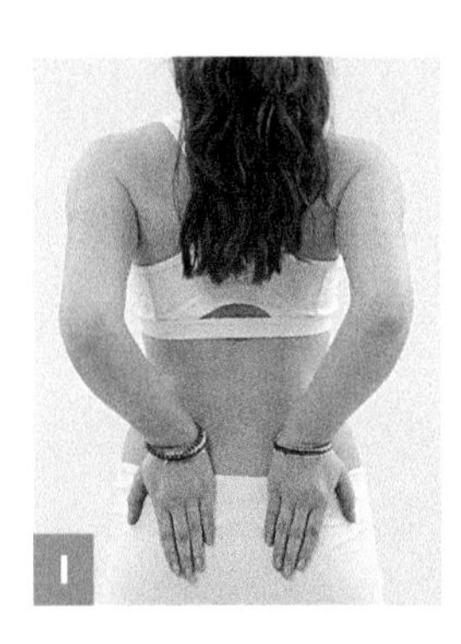


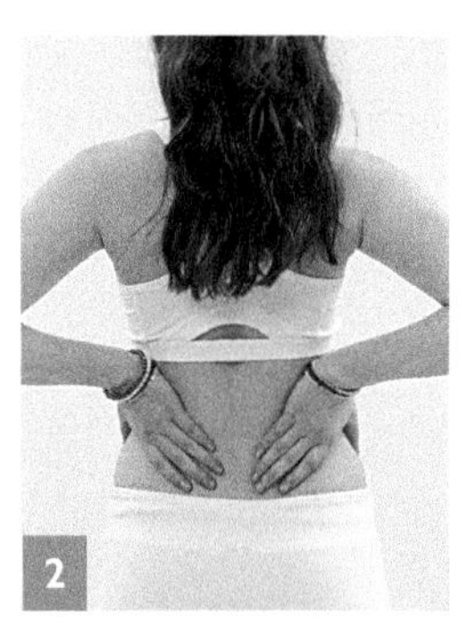


Self-treatment of the upper back is only possible to a limited extent. But you can, as described on page 135 for partner massage (points 1 to 3), treat the lower back. Stand or sit upright to reach the Marmas on the buttocks and lower back (photo **1**).

Then place your hands in a Mudra on the back and the kidneys (photo **2**). The fingertips lie on the sacroiliac joints and their Marmas.

## Treatment of the chest Marmas

**Effects:** Strengthens the respiratory organs and the heart, has a soothing effect on the chest organs in coughs, colds, bronchial asthma, grief and sorrow, nervous disorders and anxiety that are located in the chest. Enlivens and refreshes all organs of the body, is effective in fatigue, back pain, impaired concentration, waning memory. Strengthens the back (Avalambaka), the nervous system (Tarpaka), the organs of elimination (Apana), heart and circulation (Vyana, Sadhaka). Harmonizes intestinal peristalsis (Samana), strengthens the digestive fire (Pachaka, Ranjaka) and balances all three Doshas.

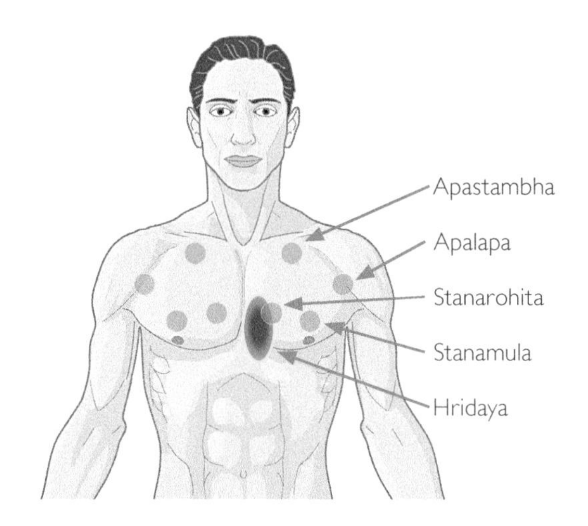


*Overview of chest Marmas*

**Oils:** For relaxation and calming: Vata massage oil, rose, sesame or almond oil; for strengthening heart energy: hawthorn blossom oil; for opening the respiratory tract: pine, basil, eucalyptus or camphor.

**Adhimarma:** Adiprana, Udana, Hridaya.

**Treatment time:** 5–15 minutes.

## Self-treatment

Sit upright or lie comfortably. Self-treatment is very pleasant and healing both with and without oil.

1. Circular massage of the great heart Marma (see page 77). Place your left hand on the stomach with the palm on the navel Marma. With your right hand move gently clockwise over the sternum in an oval shape.

2. Circular massage with the fingers flat over Apastambha (page 79). The two Marmas are above the ribs, left and right of the sternum, approximately at the level of the middle of its upper third.

3. Circular massage with the flat fingers or thumb over Stanarohita (page 78). The two points are closer to the sternum, left and right of it above the pectoral muscle, at about the height of the middle of the sternum.

4. Circular massage with the flat hand on Stanamula (page 78). The centre of the palm is over the nipple.

**Treatment format:** 1–3–5–7 (see page 34); repeat several times according to your preference.

## Partner treatment

The partner treatment is similar to self-treatment with the exception of point 4, Stanamula, where the massage goes around the nipple. Your partner lies comfortably and relaxed on their back, preferably on a massage table. Stand or sit comfortably to the right of him or her. First, apply some oil on the sternum.

**Contact:** The left hand is placed over the forehead, Sthapani Marma, with the right over the heart.

1. Treatment of the great heart Marma
2. Treatment of Apastambha
3. Local treatment of Stanarohita
4. Massage of Stanamula

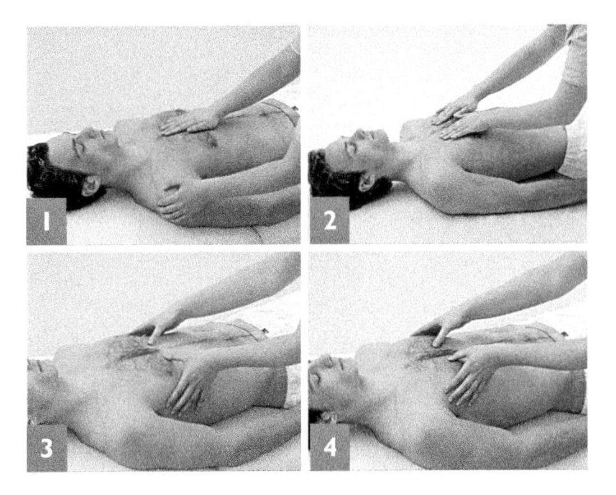

## Treatment of the 15 Marmas of the moon

Ancient palm scriptures of Siddha medicine in South India describe the influence of the moon and its various phases on the Marmas. It lists 15 main Marmas that are charged and discharged by the moon during the so-called Tithis (lunar day) in a defined sequence (a lunar month has 30 Tithis: 15 in the waxing and 15 in the waning moon). However, until now this knowledge has been hidden and the deeper aspects are still kept secret. The treatment of moon Marmas on the appropriate day is, according to tradition, said to increase sexual energy.

### Waxing and waning moon

The first half of the lunar cycle begins on the first day after the new moon, in men on the right big toe, then it moves day by day and Marma by Marma up along the right leg, continues along the midline of the body (linea alba), upwards over the neck, up to the head, and it ends at the full moon on the skull roof, the Adhipati Marma. The second cycle of the now waning moon encompasses the Marmas in reverse order, from the head over the neck and the midline of the body, back over the left leg and down to the left big toe, where it ends on the new moon.

The order is reversed in women: it starts at the left and ends at the right big toe.

### Each moon Marma has its own special quality

Each day, starting with the first day after the new moon, the focus falls on a particular Marma. If we give attention to it on that day, then it unfolds its best and most complete qualities. Each of these moon Marmas becomes blessed in a special way and fulfils specific functions in our physiology. If we treat it on the appropriate moon day, this may even help to fulfil specific aspirations. Or we can use its support for the treatment of weaknesses in our body. On the 10th and 20th day of its cycle, for example, the moon has a more powerful effect on the neck and throat Marmas and therefore on the voice, lymph organs of the throat and the thyroid. When we treat the neck and throat Marmas on these days, the treatment will be especially soothing and healing.

### Treat the moon Marmas yourself

Carry out an experiment and, for one month, monitor the effects of self-treatment of these particular moon points on their lunar day. Take 3 to 5 minutes for each point and use the 1–3–5–7 format (see page 34). Use an oil that suits you on the day or that fits best to the character of the Marma. Briefly review the list of moon Marmas in the diagram. Except for the solar plexus, which you can treat like the navel Marma, all Marmas are listed in detail, beginning on page 41. The point in the middle of the thigh may be massaged like Ani Marma.

## THE 15 MOON MARMAS AND THEIR LOCATIONS

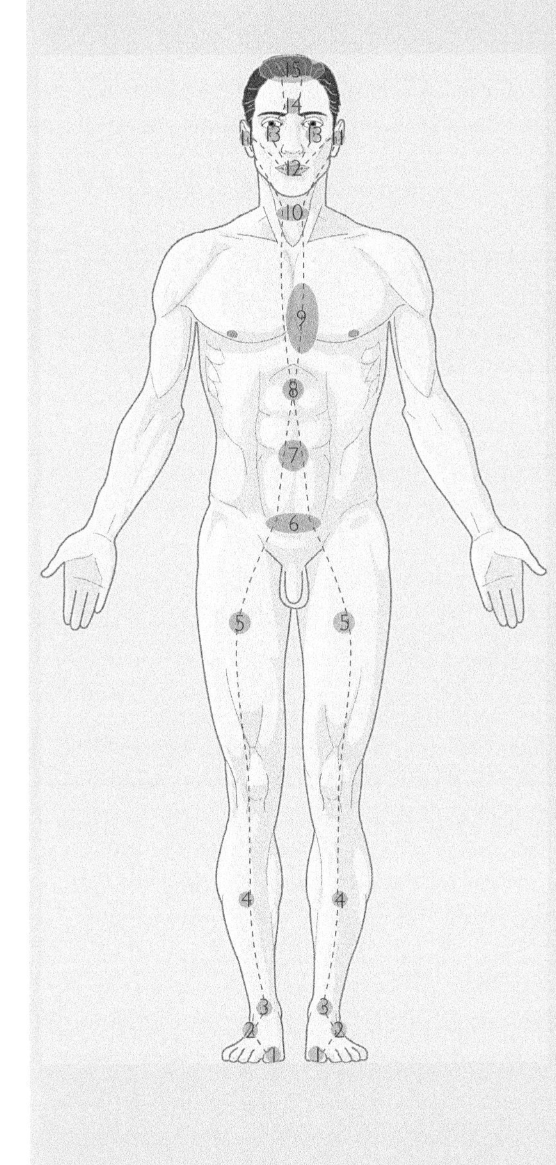


### New moon – waxing moon

**1st day after new moon** Marma of the big toe

**2nd day** Talahridaya on the top of the foot

**3rd day** Gulpha

**4th day** Counterpoint of Indrabasti on the front of the shinbone

**5th day** In the middle of the thigh – Amai Marma (Siddha name)

**6th day** Basti

**7th day** Nabhi

**8th day** Solar plexus point – Urumi Marma (Siddha name)

**9th day** Hridaya

**10th day** Pit of the throat, junction point of Nila/Manya

**11th day** Marma in front of the right ear – the front Vidhura

**12th day** Palate – Shringataka

**13th day** Under the right eye – one of the eye points

**14th day** Third eye – Sthapani

**15th day Full moon** The highest point on the skull roof – Adhipati

### Full moon – waning moon

**16th day** Third eye – Sthapani

**17th day** Under the left eye – one of the eye points

**18th day** Palate – Shringataka

**19th day** In front of the left ear – the front Vidhura

**20th day** Pit of the throat, junction point of Nila/Manya

**21st day** Hridaya

**22nd day** Solar plexus – Urumi Marma

**23rd day** Nabhi

**24th day** Basti

**25th day** In the middle of the left thigh – Amai Marma

**26th day** Counterpoint to Indrabasti on the front of the shinbone

**27th day** Gulpha

**28th day** Talahridaya on the top of the foot

**29th day** Marma of the big toe

**30th day New moon**

# Further Reading and Useful Addresses

## Ayurveda

K. L. Bhishagratna (English Translation)
*The Sushruta Samhita, Volume II*
Chowkhamba Sanskrit Series Office, Varanasi, 1991

Dr Hari Sharma
*Awakening Nature's Healing Intelligence*
Lotus Press, Twin Lakes, WI, 1998

Dr Hari Sharma
*Ayurvedic Healing: Contemporary Maharishi Ayurveda Medicine and Science*
Singing Dragon, London and Philadelphia, 2011

Dr Vasant Lad
*Textbook of Ayurveda, Volume 1: Fundamental Principles of Ayurveda*
The Ayurvedic Press, Albuquerque, New Mexico, 2002

## Meditation and Yoga

Norman E Rosenthal
*Transcendence: Healing and Transformation Through Transcendental Meditation*
Hay House UK Ltd, London, 2012

Andre Van Lysebeth and C Congreve
*Yoga Self-taught*
Red Wheel/Weiser LLC, Newburyport, MS, 2000

## Aromatherapy

Kurt Schnaubelt, PhD
*The Healing Intelligence of Essential Oils: The Science of Advanced Aromatherapy*
Healing Arts Press, Rochester, VT, 2011

## Music Therapy

Maharishi Gandharva-Ved Music
www.maharishi.co.uk/about-maharishi-gandharva-ved-music

## Veda and the Human Physiology

Dr Tony Nader, MD, PhD
*Human Physiology: Expression of Veda and the Vedic Literature*
Maharishi Vedic University, Vlodrop, 2001

## Mudras

Cain Carroll and Revital Carroll
*Mudras of India: A Comprehensive Guide to the Hand Gestures of Yoga and Indian Dance*
Singing Dragon, London and Philadelphia, 2013

## Marmas

Dr David Frawley, Dr Subhash Ranade and Dr Avinash Lele
*Ayurveda and Marma Therapy*
Lotus Press, Twin Lakes, Wisconsin, 2003

Harish Johari
*Ayurvedic Massage*
Healing Arts Press, Rochester, VT, 1996

Raakhee Mehra
*Significance of Ayurvediya Marma*
Readworthy Publications, New Delhi, 2008

## Ayurveda Products

Maharishi Ayurveda Products
Beacon House
Willow Walk
Skelmersdale
Lancashire WN8 6UR
United Kingdom
Tel: +44 1695 51015, Fax: +44 1695 50917
map@maharishi.co.uk
www.maharishi.co.uk

## Marma Oils, Aroma Oils and Sukshma Posters

Please see example poster below.
Oshadhi Ltd
Unit 6
Sycamore Close
Cambridge CB1 8PG
United Kingdom
Tel: +44 (0) 1223 242 242
info@oshadhi.co.uk
www.oshadhi.co.uk

## Marma Courses

### International

Sukshma Marma Therapy
http://sukshmamarma.org

### Germany

Deutsche Ayurveda Akademie GmbH
Steyrerweg 11, D- 93049 Regensburg
Germany
Tel: +49 (0) 941 297 080
info@ayurveda-seminare.de
www.ayurveda-seminare.de

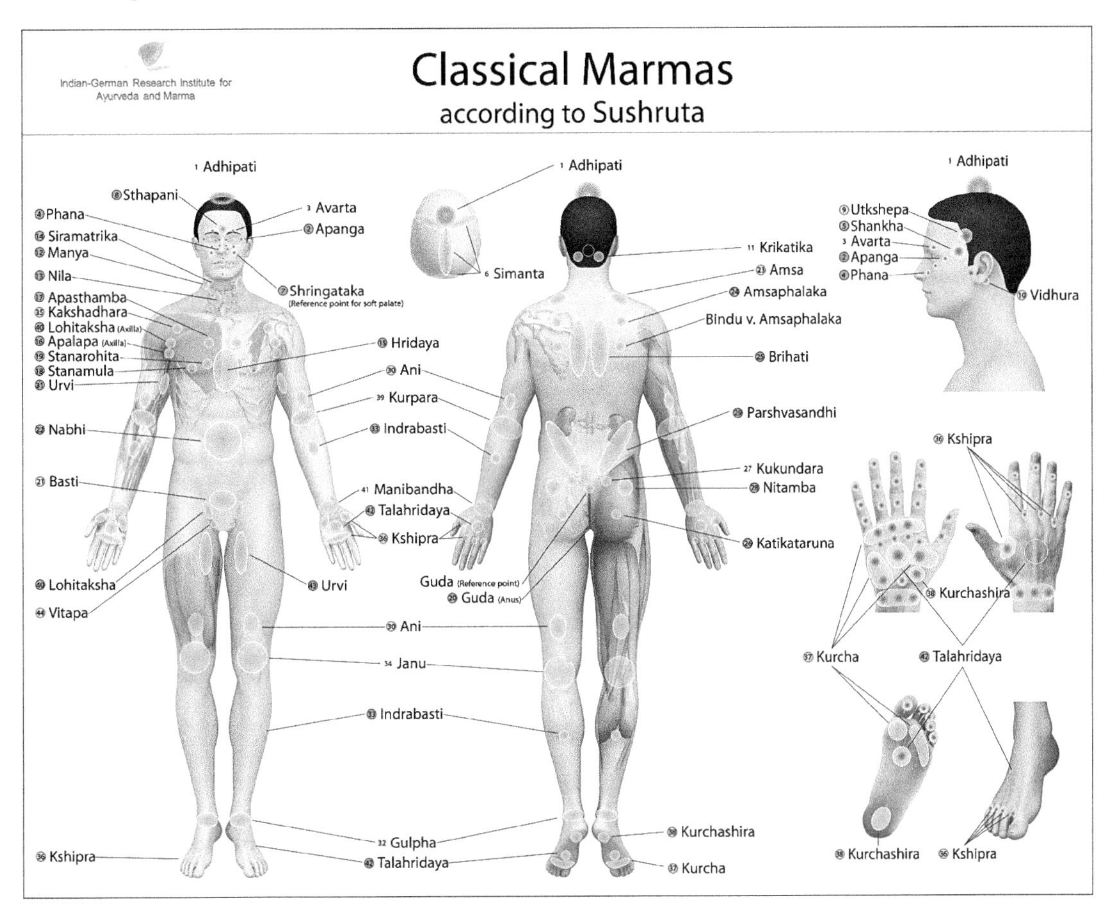

# Index

abdominal cramp 74
Adhimarma oils 37
Adhipati oil 37
Adhiprana oil 96
aggression 52
Agni 20
Ahajana (ointment on a Marma) 24
Ajna Chakra 81, 104
Ajowan oil 36
Akasha (space element) 114
almond oil 62
Alochaka 54, 91, 94, 115, 116
Ama 20
analytical intelligence 15
Ani (upper arm Marma) 54, 66
anise oil 37, 96
Anjali Mudra 77, 111, 120
anxiety 25, 56, 60, 64, 70, 74
Apana (subdosha) 12, 17, 52, 56, 60, 62, 67, 70, 72, 82, 100, 116, 134
arm pain 44, 50, 51, 52, 66, 86, 133
Arnica oil 37, 88
aromatherapy 10, 36, 37
arthritis 37, 48, 56, 60, 64
arthrosis 37, 48, 54, 56, 60, 64
Asana 30, 120f.
Asthi (bone tissue) 22, 48, 86, 100
Asthi Marma 22, 120
Atma (the Self) 11, 13, 14, 76, 91, 118
autonomic dysfunction in the neck 92
autonomic nervous system 130, 131
Avalambaka 44, 48, 56, 76, 82, 84, 115, 117, 118, 134, 136
Ayurveda 8f., 15, 26f.

back pain 48, 52, 84, 134, 136
Bala (vitality) 115, 117
basil oil 37, 96, 104, 136
Bhujangasana (cobra) 124
biliary pain 56, 64, 100
Bindu (central point) 14
bioregulators 11, 16, 17, 19, 113
biorhythm 131
bladder diseases 72
bladder weakness 50, 128
blissful joy oil 37
blocked nose 94, 100
Bodhaka 44, 92, 100
Brahmasthan 68, 74
Brahmi oil 37, 60, 64, 84, 86, 102, 106, 108
breathing exercise 30
bronchial asthma 44, 48, 52, 56, 136
bronchial infections 76
bronchitis 132
bronchospasm in asthma 44, 48, 52

Calamus oil 37
calf cramps 56
calf pain 62
calf tightness 62
Camphor oil 37, 136
carpal tunnel syndrome 48, 55
Cedar oil 37
cerebral cortex 100
cervical vertebrae, blockage of 96, 98
chest disease 76
chest pain 52
Chhandas 11
chrysanthemum oil 37
cinnamon oil 37, 46, 58, 131
circular massage 33
circulation disorders 46, 58
circulatory disorders of the head 92
circulatory insufficiency 106
circulatory weakness 50, 54, 66, 106
clove oil 37, 55
coconut oil 36, 37
colds and respiratory disorders 44, 56
colon problems 72
colour therapy 24
comfrey oil 37, 55, 88
coming back to the Self Mudra 118
confused thinking 108
consciousness 9, 10, 14, 18, 20, 26, 28, 30
constipation 132
contemplation 24, 76, 111, 114, 116, 120, 122, 128, 131
coriander oil 37
cosmic switchboard 10
cough 52, 84, 132, 136
cramping, stomach and intestinal 50, 74
crohn's disease 74
crown Chakra 102, 106, 108

deafness 96
defective vision 54, 66, 104
depression 44, 52, 104
Devata 11, 15
Dhanurasana (bow) 125
Dhatus (tissues) 11, 19, 35, 42
digestive fire 20, 42, 50, 62, 74, 86, 102, 114, 116
digestive weakness 50, 58, 66
discomfort in the neck 88
discouragement 84
disease of the pelvic organs 60
diseases of the lungs 84
diseases of the sex organs 70, 72
disorders of the salivary glands 54, 92
distributive massage 32
disturbance of vision 94
dizziness 100
Doshas 11, 15, 17, 19, 28, 34, 37, 112, 113
draining or energy-building massage 32
dry mouth 92

ear pain 96
elimination disorders of the colon 70
elimination disorders of the urinary tract 70
emotional intelligence 14
emotional relief (sadhaka) oil
energy, flow of 20, 24, 32, 50, 52, 62, 64, 98, 121
enthusiasm 117
enuresis in children 133
essential oils 10, 37
eucalyptus oil 37, 96, 104, 136
Even Temper oil (emotional Pitta disorders) 37, 77
excessive concentration 104
exhaustion 44, 70, 72
eye strain 60
eyes, overstrained 94, 100
eyes, tired 62
eyesight, strengthening 94

fatigue 48, 50, 106, 108, 114
fear 60, 64, 74, 88, 90, 94, 96, 98, 104, 117, 130, 133
fear of failure 70
fear, existential 70
feelings of peace 49, 64, 75, 76, 104, 108, 116
fennel oil 37, 74
flatulence 72, 74
fontanelle 108
foot and leg cramp 56
frankincense oil 37, 44

gall bladder ailments 64
Gandhari Nadi 91
Gandharva music 29, 39, 46, 112, 131
gastrointestinal disorders 50, 52, 92, 116
gem light therapy 24
general joint pain 37, 48
geranium oil 37
ghee (clarified butter)
ginger oil 37, 131
grief 46, 58, 84, 92, 104, 130, 131, 136
Gulpha (ankle Marma) 22, 60
Gunas 20
Gyan Mudra 114
gynaecological problems 62

haemorrhoids 62, 70
Hakini Mudra 75, 103
happiness, feelings of 108
headache 8, 25, 88, 94, 98, 99, 100, 104, 106, 132
headache in the forehead 104
headache in the temples 100, 132
headache originating from the back of the neck 88, 98, 132
headache resulting from strained eyes 94, 100
hearing and smell 102
heart disorders, nervous 46, 52, 56
heart disorders, organic and vegetative 76, 84
heart disorders, psychological 84
heart failure 84
heart palpitations 130
heat in the legs 131
heavenly peace massage oil 37
heavy tongue, feeling of 92
hepatobiliary disorders 64
herbal and mineral supplements 24
herbal teas 24
high blood pressure 76
hip pain 67, 72
hoarse voice 116
hoarseness 92, 132
hormonal disorders 54, 66
hot stone therapy 24, 27
Hridaya oil 37, 46, 48, 58, 60, 76, 84, 86, 100, 130, 131, 136

Ida Nadi 80, 90
impotence 70
indigestion 46, 50, 74, 86, 92
indigestion in colon and small intestine 92
indigestion in stomach 92
Indra 50
Indra Royal oil
Indrabasti (forearm and calf Marma) 22, 50, 62, 72, 122, 132, 138
inner restlessness 64, 74
inner settledness 48
inner tension 84
insecurity, mental and physical 60
insomnia 25, 104, 106, 108
intestinal inflammation 74
intuition 108
irritable bladder 72

Janu (knee Marma) 64, 128, 130, 133
Janu Sirasana (sitting forward bend) 122, 124
jasmine oil 37, 46, 70, 72, 74, 76, 86, 88, 106
jewellery 24, 97
joint soothe oil 37, 52, 53, 54, 56, 64, 66, 67, 98
jojoba oil 36, 37
juniper oil 37, 54

Kakshadhara (shoulder muscle Marma) 55, 67, 122
Kalari 10, 21, 33
Kalari Payat 21
Kalari Payirchi 21
Kapha aroma oil 37, 44,
Kapha massage oil 37, 44, 96
Kati Basti 27
kidney disease 54, 58, 66, 133
knee injury 64
knee pain 64, 133
kneecap pain (chondropathia patellae) 64
Kshipra (Marmas between the fingers and the toes) 44, 45, 56, 92, 94, 96, 112, 114, 116, 128, 133
Kurcha and Kurchashira (heel of the hand Marmas and equivalent on the foot) 54, 66, 70, 114, 115, 116
Kurpara (elbow Marma) 52, 122, 128, 130
lack of confidence 84
lack of coordination in walking 60
lassi 24
lavender 28
lavender oil 37, 48, 56, 60, 64, 86, 100, 131
lemon oil 37, 84, 134
lemongrass oil 37, 84, 134
Lepam 24
life or Prana Mudra 115
liver and bile problems 64
liver and gallbladder disease 56
Lohitaksha (Marma of the armpit and groin) 20, 44, 55, 56, 67, 115, 117, 122, 125, 133
longitudinal strokes 33, 36, 89, 135
loss of balance in life 74
lotus oil 37, 46, 70, 72, 76, 104, 106,
lung and bronchial disease 84
lymphedema in legs 62

MA 628 joint oil 37, 50, 52, 54, 55, 56, 60, 64, 84, 88, 96
MA 634 mint oil 37, 44, 56
magnesium 130
Mahabhutas (virtual elements) 34, 113
Mahaojas oil 37, 48, 52
Maharishi Ayurveda 37, 140, 141
Maharishi Mahesh Yogi 10
Maharishi Patanjali 120
Mamsa Marma 22, 46, 50, 58, 62, 70
Manibandha (the wrist Marma) 13, 18, 48, 49, 122, 128, 130, 131, 132, 133
marjoram oil 37
Marma oils 37
Marmadhara 24
martial art 10, 21, 33
Matsyendrasana (half spinal twist) 122, 125
medicinal waters 24
meditation 8, 10, 24, 30, 77, 102, 112, 114, 116, 120, 126, 130, 131, 132, 141
menopause 54, 133
menstrual disorders 70, 72, 133
menstrual pain 133
mental dullness 62
mental fatigue 48, 50
mental overexertion 100
mental relaxation 115
mental restlessness 60, 64
mental stress 106
metals 24
milk compress 132
mint oil 37, 62, 100, 104
moon 9, 14, 35, 102, 138, 139

MP16 Nasya oil 132
Mudra 24, 30, 45, 49, 61, 65, 75, 77, 85, 103, 104, 106, 108, 110 – 118, 130, 131, 133, 136
myrrh oil 37

Nabhi oil 37, 58, 60, 64, 74, 86
Nadis of colon and lungs 112
Nakshatra (lunar mansion) 14
narrow-mindedness 104
nasal congestion 100
naturopathic medicine 25
nausea 100
neck tension 44, 51, 88, 89, 93, 98, 106, 132
nervous disorders 72, 136
nervous disorders of the heart 130
nervous heart complaints 46, 52, 56, 58, 76, 79, 104
nervous weakness 70, 102
nervousness 25, 46, 48, 58, 64, 104, 106, 108
Netri Marma 104
Nidra Marma oil 37, 48
nutmeg oil 37

Ojas 19, 20, 26, 34, 50, 68, 76, 78, 102, 108, 105, 117, 130
orange oil 37, 134
Oshadhi 37
overstrained eyes 104

Pachaka 46, 48, 50, 52, 58, 60, 62, 74, 86, 134, 136
pain in general 44
pain in the back 48, 51, 52, 56, 62, 66, 72, 134
pain in the big toe 56
pain in the knee 64
pain in the neck 48, 51, 52, 55, 88, 98, 99, 133
pain in the shoulder 44, 52
pain or tension in the foot 58
Pandits 30
paralysis and numbness in the arm 86
partner treatment 8, 32, 34
Payasvini Nadi 91
peristaltic movement 116
pine oil 37, 96, 136
pineal gland 108
Pingala Nadi 80, 90, 91, 122
Pitta aroma oil 37, 58, 92
Pitta massage oil 37, 48, 58, 92, 94
Pitta oil 36, 66
pituitary gland 54, 104, 122
Prana 4, 10, 14, 30, 33, 35, 42, 43
Prana Mudra 115
Pranayama 24, 32,126, 129, 130, 131, 133
primordial sound 9, 10
prostate diseases 70
prostate problems 62, 66, 72
psychological heart disease 84
Pusha Nadi 91

raisin water 130
Rajas 19, 20
Ranjaka 52, 60, 74, 134, 136
Rasa 26, 76, 83,
Rasayanas 24, 26
reflexology zone 44, 113, 115, 134
regeneration 118, 126
rejuvenation 8, 26
respiratory diseases 114
respiratory tract 52
restless leg syndrome 60, 133
restlessness 46, 56, 58, 60, 64, 74
rhinitis 100
rings 24
Rishi 11, 15
root Chakra 91, 115, 117, 122, 124
rose oil 37, 48, 70, 72, 74, 76, 84, 94, 100, 104, 130, 136
rose water 95, 105, 133
rosemary oil 37, 48
rosewood oil 37, 84

Sadhaka pitta 17, 44, 46, 48, 52, 56, 58, 62, 76, 84, 100, 104, 114, 118
saffron oil 50, 104
Sahasrara Chakra 81, 106, 108
saliva, excess flow of 92
Samana 12, 62, 74, 82, 116, 118, 134, 136
Samvahana (enlivening exercise) 123
sandalwood oil 37, 50, 72, 74, 76, 88, 94, 104, 132
sandalwood paste 132
Sandhi Marma 22, 48, 52, 60, 64, 83, 94, 98, 106
Sangam 18, 44, 112, 114
Sarvangasana (shoulder stand) 124
Sattva 19, 20
Savasana (resting position) 126
sciatica 62, 122
self-confidence 76, 77, 84, 85, 118, 122, 124, 130, 133
self-confidence, strengthening 76, 104
self-discovery 120
sense of taste 92, 102
senses, overstimulation of the 52, 131
sesame oil 36, 37, 70, 72, 74, 108, 134
sexual disorders 60, 62, 70, 72
sexual weakness 50, 66, 70
Shalabhasana (locust) 125
Shankhini Nadi 91
shoulder and arm pain 52, 86
shoulder pain 44, 98, 133
Shukra (reproductive tissue) 60, 115, 116
silence in consciousness 120
singing bowls 24
Sira (vessel) 22,
Sira Marmas 5, 74, 76, 84, 92, 93, 94, 102, 104
skin diseases 133
sleeping disorder 5, 56, 58, 60, 64, 100, 128, 131
smooth cycle oil 37
Snayu (tendon) 22
Snayu Marma 44, 56, 72, 88, 96, 100
soft palate 102
solar plexus 11, 13, 16, 76, 79, 95, 118, 138, 139
soma 102
sorrow 37, 46, 58, 76, 84, 92, 130, 131, 136
sound therapies 24
speech disturbance 92
spiced milk 131
spinal weakness and discomfort 76
spleen and pancreatic disorders 64
St Johns Wort oil 131
Sthapani oil 100, 104
stiff neck 98, 99
stimulation of lymphatic flow 44, 56
strained eyes 94, 100, 104, 132
strength 22, 35, 46, 50, 56, 58, 62, 74, 76, 82, 84, 85, 104, 108, 117
strengthening of self-confidence 76
stress-induced bowel dysfunction 48
Subdoshas 4, 17, 112, 113
sun 35, 36, 102, 114
sun or Akash Mudra 114
sunflower oil 36, 37
supervisory control unit 102
Sushruta Samhita 8, 10, 14
sutures, cranial 106
swallowing problems 92
sweet almond oil 76

Takradhara 25
Talahridaya (the heart of the hand and foot Marma) 5, 12, 13, 17, 35, 36, 42, 43, 46, 54, 58, 66, 74, 76, 77, 84, 112, 114-118, 122, 130, 131, 133, 139
Tamas 19, 20
tapping or light clapping 33

Tarpaka (subdosha) 50, 76, 84, 98, 102, 104, 106, 108, 134, 136
taste disorders 102
teeth grinding 100
tennis elbow 51, 52, 53
tension in the wrist 48
the conch shell Mudra 116
the fist Mudra 117
throat Chakra 88, 91, 92, 117
thyroid 44, 54, 66, 93, 116, 138
tinnitus 48, 60, 96, 133
tinnitus and eye strain 60
tired eyes 62
tired legs 62, 66
tonsillitis 44, 116
toothache 56
touching without massage 33
traditional Chinese medicine (TCM) 10, 13, 43, 44, 50, 62, 94, 98
transcendental meditation 30, 130, 131
trembling of the hands 52

Udana (Subdosha) 12, 37, 44, 48, 50, 56, 86, 88, 92, 98, 102, 114, 116, 131, 132, 134, 136
Udana oil 98
ulcerative colitis 74
urinary retention 56
Urvi or Bahvi (the vascular Marma on the upper arm and leg) 55, 67, 122, 133
Uttanasana (standing forward bend) 125

Vajrasana (diamond posture) 5, 122, 124
valerian oil 37, 56, 60, 64, 106, 131
Vata disorders 36, 44, 48, 128, 132
Vata massage oil 37, 44, 46, 48, 50, 52, 55, 58, 70, 72, 74, 76, 86, 88, 92, 96, 106, 130, 131, 132, 134, 136
Vata oil 56, 60, 62, 64, 98, 100, 102, 108
Vata tea 131
Vayu (air element) 114
Vayu Mudra 116
Veda 9, 10, 24, 29, 46, 91, 112, 120, 140
Vedic astrology 11, 14
Vedic music 24, 29, 46
Vedic recitation 29
Vellan (rolling) 123
Vetiver oil 37
victory Mudra 117
vigorous rubbing 33, 99
visual impairment 66, 104
vital points 6, 8, 9, 13, 18, 27, 29, 40, 64, 98
Vyana (subdosha) 12, 46, 48, 50, 52, 58, 62, 74, 76, 78, 84, 92, 106, 134, 136

warm footbath 132
weakness of concentration 48
worry 17, 104
worry free oil 76, 130, 131

Yagya (Vedic ceremony) 4, 24, 30
yoga 4, 5, 11, 24, 30, 42, 85, 87, 90, 119, 120-125, 130, 131, 132, 141
yoga sutras 120

# Acknowledgements


## From Dr. Ernst Schrott

I offer my deep gratitude and heartfelt thanks to my friends Dr. M. A. Kumar, Deputy Adviser for Siddha Medicine, Ministry of Health and Family Welfare of the Government of India, New Delhi, and Dr. T. Mohana Raj, Marma expert, author and president of the A.T. Siddha Vaidya Sangam, Munchirai, Trivandrum. They led me to the best Marma Therapy centres in South India to help me prepare this book.

Very special thanks to Dr Pavani Raju, who has a brilliant mind with deep and comprehensive understanding of the science of Marma. Many thanks also to Dr Aditya and Dr Harsha Raju. Whenever I had a question, there was always an excellent answer, mostly via Internet.

Also I would like to thank Vaidya Kalyan Chakravarthy for his advice and assistance.

Maria, my dear daughter, deserves special recognition and thanks. Despite the fact that she was preparing for her final school exams, she still managed to find time to draw the illustrations for this book.

Many thanks also to Anja and Natalia! You carried out this gentle Marma Therapy on patients in my practice with sensitivity and empathy and have therefore become the most important source of practical experience.

I would like to thank Katrina Tausch, our photo model, for her patience and perseverance. Her complexion and grace have immeasurably enriched our book.

Finally, I would like to give warm thanks and gratitude to the translator Marek Lorys. It is very fortunate that Marek is a professional translator and has also attended all my courses, so has all the knowledge of Sukshma Marma. In addition, he is a teacher of Transcendental Meditation with a background in the development of consciousness and Maharishi Ayurveda. Marek and I read through the entire book together, word by word, which has made this book a very special contribution to the practical knowledge of Marma treatment.

## From all three authors

We would particularly like to thank Maharishi Mahesh Yogi, who was the first person in our time to re-enliven Vedic knowledge and Ayurveda in their completeness. He also defined the significance of Marmas as the seat of the Veda and as connection points between man and cosmos, all in accordance with the classical Vedic texts. His greatest concern was to protect the Marmas and to treat them with utmost care.


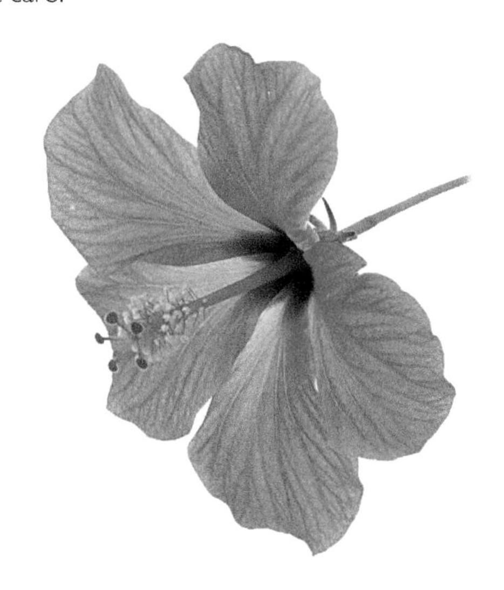

# About the authors

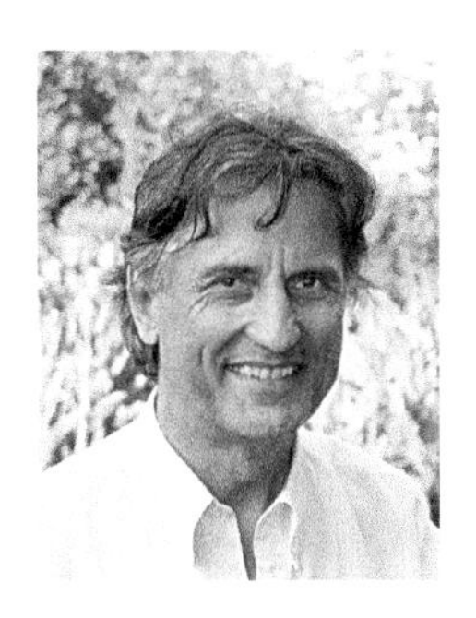

Dr. Ernst Schrott is a trained medical doctor specialised in naturopathy and homeopathy and one of the most renowned Ayurveda specialists in Germany and Europe. He is vice-president of the German Society of Ayurveda (*Deutsche Gesellschaft für Ayurveda*), head of the German Academy of Ayurveda and has written numerous bestsellers on Ayurveda.

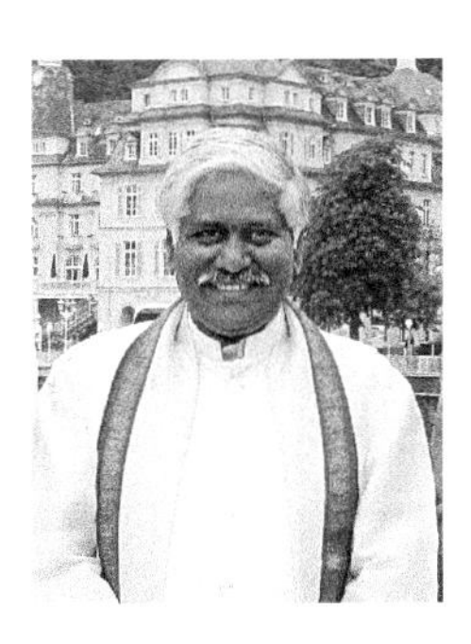

The internationally recognized Ayurveda specialist Vaidya Dr. J. Ramanuja Raju is chief physician of the Maharishi Ayurveda Clinic in New Delhi and general secretary of the All India Ayurvedic Graduate Association. He was advisor to the Indian State Ministry of Health and Family Welfare and has trained thousands of doctors in Ayurveda worldwide. He is also a master of the art of Ayurvedic pulse diagnosis.

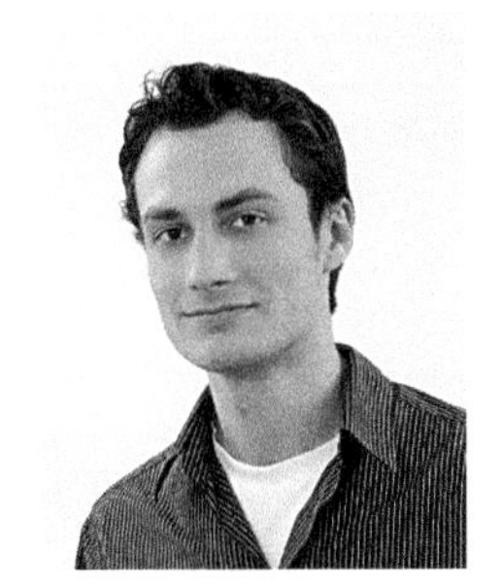

Stefan Schrott, born in 1981, studied traditional Vedic techniques of Yoga and Meditation at the Maharishi University of Management in Fairfield, Iowa. He is a holistic therapist for mind/body medicine, Maharishi Ayurveda and Marma and a certified Yoga instructor (WMYA). Inspired by Vedic healing techniques and practical training in the USA, India and Europe, he is especially devoted to spiritual healing.

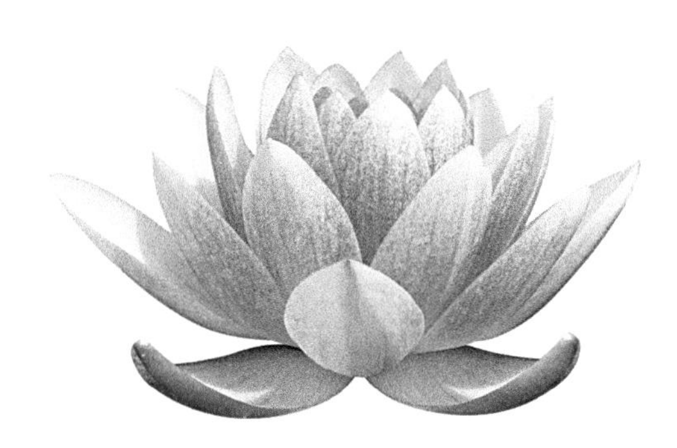